Tumors of the Nervous System

Wiley Series in Diagnostic and Therapeutic Radiology

Luther W. Brady, M.D., Editor

Professor and Chairman, Department of Therapeutic Radiology and Nuclear Medicine, Hahnemann Medical College and Hospital, Philadelphia, Pennsylvania

TUMORS OF THE NERVOUS SYSTEM

Edited by H. Gunter Seydel, M.D., M.S.

CANCER OF THE LUNG

Edited by H. Gunter Seydel, M.D., M.S.
Arnold Chait, M.D.
John T. Gmelich, M.D.

Tumors of the Nervous System

Edited by

H. Gunter Seydel, M.D., M.S.

*Associate Professor of Radiation Therapy
and Nuclear Medicine,
The Jefferson Medical College of the
Thomas Jefferson University,
Philadelphia, Pennsylvania*

*Chief, Department of Radiation Therapy,
American Oncologic Hospital of the
Fox Chase Cancer Center,
Philadelphia, Pennsylvania*

*Proceedings of the Fourth Annual Symposium
of the American Oncologic Hospital
of the Fox Chase Cancer Center*

A WILEY BIOMEDICAL-HEALTH PUBLICATION

JOHN WILEY & SONS
New York / London / Sydney / Toronto

Library of Congress Cataloging in Publication Data:

Main entry under title:
Tumors of the nervous system.

 (Wiley series in diagnostic and therapeutic radiology)
 "A Wiley biomedical-health publication."
 Includes bibliographical references and index.
 1. Nervous system—Tumors—Congresses. I. Seydel,
H. Gunter, ed. II. Philadelphia. American Oncologic Hospital.
[DNLM: 1. Acromegaly—Therapy—Congresses. 2. Brain
neoplasms—Congresses. 3. Glioma—Therapy—Congresses.
4. Pituitary neoplasms—Therapy—Congresses.

W3 C1164N 1973t / WL358 C215 1973t]
RC280.N4T85   616.9′94′8   74-26714
ISBN 0-471-77848-6

Printed in the United States of America

10 9 8 7 6 5 4 3 2 1

Authors

Antoniades, John, M.D., Associate Professor, Department of Radiation Therapy and Nuclear Medicine, Hahnemann Medical College, Philadelphia, Pennsylvania

Asbell, Sucha O., M.D., Assistant Professor, Department of Radiation Therapy and Nuclear Medicine, Hahnemann Medical College, Philadelphia, Pennsylvania

Brady, Luther W., M.D., Professor and Chairman, Department of Therapeutic Radiology and Nuclear Medicine, Hahnemann Medical College and Hospital, Philadelphia, Pennsylvania

Carmichael, Paul, M.D., Associate Surgeon, Retina Service, Wills Eye Hospital, Philadelphia, Pennsylvania

Chang, Chu H., M.D., Professor of Radiology, College of Physicians and Surgeons, Columbia University, New York, New York; Director, Division of Radiotherapy, Columbia-Presbyterian Medical Center, New York, New York

Croll, Millard N., M.D., Professor of Radiation Therapy and Nuclear Medicine, Hahnemann Medical College, Philadelphia, Pennsylvania

Ertel, Inta J., M.D., Associate Professor of Pediatrics, Ohio State University, Children's Hospital, Columbus, Ohio

Glassburn, John R., M.D., Assistant Professor, Department of Radiation Therapy and Nuclear medicine, Hahnemann Medical College, Philadelphia, Pennsylvania

Griem, Melvin L., M.D., Professor and Chairman, Division of Radiation Therapy, Chicago Tumor Institute of the University of Chicago, Chicago, Illinois

Herbert, Charles M., Jr., A. B., Associate, College of Physicians and Surgeons, Columbia University, New York, New York; Radiation Physicist, Division of Radiotherapy, Columbia-Presbyterian Medical Center, New York, New York

Housepian, Edgar M., M.D., Associate Professor of Clinical Neurological Surgery, College of Physicians and Surgeons, Columbia University, New York, New York; Associate Attending Neurological Surgeon, Neurological Institute, Columbia-Presbyterian Medical Center, New York, New York

Kjellberg, Raymond N., M.D., Associate Clinical Professor of Surgery, Harvard Medical School, Cambridge, Massachusetts; Visiting Neurosurgeon, Massachusetts General Hospital, Boston, Massachusetts

Kramer, Simon, M.D., Professor and Chairman, Department of Radiation Therapy and Nuclear Medicine, Thomas Jefferson University Hospital, Philadelphia, Pennsylvania

Lessig, Harry J., M.D., Fellow in Nuclear Medicine, Hahnemann Medical College, Philadelphia, Pennsylvania

Levin, Seymour R., M.D., Chief, Metabolic Unit, Wadsworth Veterans Administration Hospital, Los Angeles, California; Assistant Professor of Medicine, University of California, Los Angeles, California; Assistant Research Physician, Metabolic Research Unit, University of California, San Francisco, California

Mancall, Elliott L., M.D., Professor of Medicine, Director, Division of Neurology, Hahnemann Medical College, Philadelphia, Pennsylvania

Marks, J. E., M.D., American Cancer Society Junior Faculty Fellow, Division of Radiation Therapy, Chicago Tumor Institute of the University of Chicago, Chicago, Illinois

Mullan, John F., M.D., John Harper Seeley Professor and Chairman of Neurosurgery, University of Chicago Hospitals and Clinics, Chicago, Illinois

Newton, W. A., Jr., M.D., Professor of Pathology and Pediatrics, Ohio State University, Children's Hospital, Columbus, Ohio

Prasasvinichai, Sriprayoon, M.D., Assistant Professor, Department of Radiation Therapy and Nuclear Medicine, Hahnemann Medical College, Philadelphia, Pennsylvania

Sayers, M. P., M.D., Associate Professor of the Department of Surgery, Division of Neurosurgery, Ohio State University, Chief of Neurosurgery, Children's Hospital, Columbus, Ohio

Schatanoff, David, M.D., Assistant Professor, Department of Radiation Therapy and Nuclear Medicine, Hahnemann Medical College, Philadelphia, Pennsylvania

Sciarra, Daniel, M.D., Professor of Clinical Neurology, College of Physicians and Surgeons, Columbia University, New York, New York; Attending Neurologist, Neurological Institute, Columbia-Presbyterian Medical Center, New York, New York

Seydel, H. Gunter, M.D., M.S., Chief, Department of Radiation Therapy, American Oncologic Hospital of the Fox Chase Cancer Center, Philadelphia, Pennsylvania; Associate Professor of Radiation Therapy and Nuclear Medicine, The Jefferson Medical College, The Thomas Jefferson University, Philadelphia, Pennsylvania

Sheline, Glenn E., Ph.D., M.D., Professor of Radiology, Section of Radiation Oncology, University of California, San Francisco, California

Steward, William, M.D., Professor of Radiology, University of Chicago, Director of Chicago Tumor Institute, Chicago, Illinois

Torpie, Richard J., M.D., Assistant Professor, Department of Radiation Therapy and Nuclear Medicine, Hahnemann Medical College, Philadelphia, Pennsylvania

Wadwa, Janak, M.D., Clinical Assistant Professor of Pediatrics, Ohio State University, Children's Hospital, Columbus, Ohio

Wallner, Robert J., D.O., Assistant Professor of Radiation Therapy and Nuclear Medicine, Hahnemann Medical College, Philadelphia, Pennsylvania

Wara, William M., M.D., Assistant Professor of Radiation Oncology, University of California, San Francisco Medical Center, San Francisco, California

Yung, Wai-Kwan, B.Sc., American Cancer Society Student Fellow, Illinois Division, Chicago, Illinois

Preface

We continue to be proud of the increased interest shown in the Annual Cancer Symposium held on the campus of the Fox Chase Cancer Center. Each year, attendance figures indicate that physicians welcome the opportunity to achieve continuing education in current diagnosis and treatment of cancer and to engage in a fruitful discussion with outstanding speakers. We desire to provide information on new approaches that can serve practicing physicians in the care of their cancer patients.

The current symposium confronts the problems of neoplasia of the nervous system. Rapid dissemination of new knowledge gained from basic and clinical research will allow the attending physicians to return to their practice with a useful picture of research activities applicable to the treatment of patients with tumors of the nervous system. The program would not be possible without the help of an outstanding list of guest speakers representing basic science, diagnosis, and therapy.

We extend our thanks to the Philadelphia Division of the American Cancer Society, the Applied Radiation Corporation, the Atomic Energy of Canada, Ltd., Corporation, E. R. Squibb & Sons, Inc., and Merck, Sharp & Dohme for their support in making this symposium possible.

This volume was prepared for publication with the support of The American Oncologic Hospital by the following members of the Department of Radiation Therapy: Rose Hoffman, Kathleen Secoda, Rose Marie Miller and Anita Shapiro.

H. Gunter Seydel

September 1974
Philadelphia, Pennsylvania

Contents

Tumors of the Nervous System

Introduction

H. Gunter Seydel, M.D., M.S.,
Chief, Department of Radiation Therapy,
American Oncologic Hospital of the
Fox Chase Cancer Center,
Philadelphia, Pennsylvania;
Associate Professor of Radiation
Therapy and Nuclear Medicine,
The Jefferson Medical College,
Thomas Jefferson University,
Philadelphia, Pennsylvania

Tumors of the brain and cranial meninges represent a relatively small percentage of all human tumors. The Third National Cancer Survey[3] indicated that the age-adjusted incidence rate for males in the United States was 5.3 per 100,000, and for females 3.7 per 100,000. The report *Cancer Mortality and Morbidity Pennsylvania*[1] published by the Department of Health of the Commonwealth of Pennsylvania has shown that the relative incidence was 1.6% of all cancers in Pennsylvania. There was no significant change in this relative incidence between 1958 and 1971. The cancer morbidity in Pennsylvania in 1971 was approximately 250 per 100,000 population, indicating that approximately 500 patients are diagnosed as having tumors of the nervous system in our state every year. For the United States as a whole, approximately 9000 patients may be expected to develop such tumors yearly.

A striking feature of the treatment of tumors of the brain and cranial meninges is the poor survival rate in spite of their classification as "localized disease" in the national survey of the End Results Group of the National Cancer Institute.[2] Only 40% of the patients diagnosed as having cancer of the brain or cranial meninges survived more than 1 year after diagnosis. A 3-year survival of 28% was found for the years 1940–1949, which increased to 37% for the years 1965–1969. The percentage of patients diagnosed with "localized disease" increased from 71% for the period 1940–1949 to 80% for the period 1955–1969. Surgery remains the most effective treatment; however, only 48% of the reported patients could be treated in this manner. The 1-year survival of patients treated by surgery was 45% if localized disease was present, with a 3-year survival of 42%.

Improvements in results of treatment of many malignancies have been quite striking in the last decade, but the treatment of cancer of the brain and cranial meninges remains by and large disappointing. New avenues of treatment in the form of a combination of surgery, radiation therapy, and chemotherapy are being explored in cooperative studies such as the Brain Tumor Study Group and the Radiation Therapy Oncology Group of the National Cancer Institute. It is expected that over the next 5 to 10 years significant information will be received from these cooperative trials, and there is reason to believe that an improvement in the prognosis of the patient diagnosed as having cancer of the nervous system might emerge.

REFERENCES

1. Cancer Mortality and Morbidity Pennsylvania, Commonwealth of Pennsylvania, Department of Health, Harrisburg, Pennsylvania, 1972.
2. End Results in Cancer. Report No. 4. U.S. Department of Health, Education and Welfare, National Cancer Institute, Bethesda, Maryland, 1972.
3. Preliminary Report, Third National Cancer Survey, 1969 Incidence. Department of Health, Education and Welfare Publication, No. (NIH) 72-128, Washington, D.C., 1971.

The Use of Radionuclides in the Diagnosis of Tumors of the Central Nervous System

Millard M. Croll, M.D.,

Professor of Radiation Therapy
and Nuclear Medicine,
Hahnemann Medical College,
Philadelphia, Pennsylvania

Robert J. Wallner, D.O.,

Assistant Professor of Radiation
Therapy and Nuclear Medicine,
Hahnemann Medical College,
Philadelphia, Pennsylvanis

Paul Carmichael, M.D.,

Associate Surgeon,
Retina Service,
Wills Eye Hospital,
Philadelphia, Pennsylvania

Harry J. Lessig, M.D.,

Fellow in Nuclear Medicine,
Hahnemann Medical College,
Philadelphia, Pennsylvania

Procedures for noninvasive diagnosis of central nervous system tumors range from the lumbar puncture and skull roentgenogram to the formidable contrast radiological studies. The use of radionuclide tracer techniques has had a major impact on neurodiagnosis. The nuclear medicine modality has unquestionably altered neurologic and neurosurgical practice and has contributed immeasurably to care. This chapter deals with the use of radionuclides in four major areas: static imaging of the brain, functional studies of the cerebral circulation, evaluation of cerebrospinal fluid dynamics, and tracer techniques for detection and localization of intraocular and intraorbital tumors.

BRAIN TUMOR LOCALIZATION WITH RADIONUCLIDES

The detection and localization of neoplastic lesions in the brain as well as detection of nonneoplastic lesions with radioactive materials should properly be called *radionuclidic cephaloscintigraphy,* but the original term of "brain scanning" has remained. The brain is a most susceptible organ for external measurement and detection of a gamma-emitting radionuclide. Prior to the development of brain scanning, a gap existed between the neurodiagnostic procedures of skull roentgenography and electroencephalography and the potentially hazardous arteriography with contrast media. Thus, brain scanning has gained widespread acceptance because of its safety and lack of morbidity and mortality, and is now recognized as an accurate neurodiagnostic screening procedure. This modality elicits direct evidence and visualization of a tumor since the radionuclide localizes within the lesion complex. This compares to the presumptive and indirect evidence presented by the neuroradiologic contrast procedures that become positive through the displacement of normal intracranial structures. The exact localization of a cerebral space-occupying lesion can be of great value when neurosurgical procedures are undertaken.

Indications

Brain imaging is indicated in the following situations:[8]

1. All patients suspected of having a space-occupying lesion.
2. Evaluation of patients following the diagnosis of a primary lesion known to be associated with intracranial metastasis.
3. Serial examination of patients with CNS malignancy following neurosurgery, chemotherapy, or radiation therapy.
4. Patients with focal neurological signs—particularly those indicating hemispherical involvement (i.e., unilateral weakness, speech disturbance, homonymous field defect). The presence of homonymous hemianopsia may be considered an absolute indication.
5. Patients with significant (i.e., focal) electroencephalographic abnormalities.
6. Patients with epilepsy of late onset.

Radiopharmaceuticals and Mechanism of Localization

The history of radiopharmaceuticals for brain imaging is rapid but extensive. Thirty-five years ago Duran-Reynals[1] reported the localization of various organic dyes and

7

foreign proteins in tumors. He found a significant difference between concentration of the dyes in the normal brain and concentration in tumors. This was confirmed by the use of fluorescein[2] 8 years later and at that time ^{32}P was also used to localize tumors at surgery.[3] The first labeled material was ^{131}I-tagged diiodofluorescein in 1948.[4] This was followed in 1951 by ^{131}I serum albumin,[5] which proved to be reasonably successful. Many other substances such as ^{74}As and ^{64}Cu were utilized, but the first major breakthrough occurred in the late 1950s when Blau and Bender[6] developed ^{203}Hg-labeled chlormerodrin. The next major breakthrough occurred in 1964 with the introduction of technetium-99m pertechnetate.[7] This radionuclide continues to be the most popular agent because of its ideal physical properties for scanning and widespread availability.

Pertechnetate is thought to localize in CNS tumors secondary to a breakdown in the blood–brain barrier that corresponds to the capillary endothelium. Normally, the intercellular spaces are in close approximation causing retention of radionuclide within the circulation.

In the presence of a very vascular tumor the increase in blood volume alone is sufficient to cause increased isotope localization. Neovascularity in tumors is associated with abnormal intercellular junctions that are semipermeable, allowing radionuclide leakage into adjunct tissues. When edema is present the increase in extracellular fluid (particularly in the presence of a high protein content) interferes with cell approximation and causes an associated increase in isotope concentration. Only rarely will ^{99m}Tc localize within the tumor cell itself (possibly secondary to the mechanism of pinocytosis) and then usually in quantities that are insufficient for imaging purposes.

There has been interest in the detection of CNS tumors utilizing radionuclides considered to be tumor-specific. Gallium-67 citrate was the first agent to be investigated for this purpose.[9] ^{67}Ga was found to localize in both primary intracranial neoplasms [e.g., glioblastoma multiforme and meningiomas (Figs. 4c and 4d)] and in metastatic lesions. It may be useful in differentiating tumor from infarction and in separating the presence of tumor recurrence from postneurosurgical changes visualized on the routine pertechnetate scan.

More recently attention has been focused on the use of bleomycin labeled with ^{99m}Tc, ^{111}In, and ^{57}Co in the detection of intracranial neoplasms.[10] Bleomycin is an antibiotic that acts as an oncostatic polypeptide demonstrating a high affinity for potentially malignant tumors, especially squamous cell carcinoma. It demonstrates rapid plasma clearance, permitting a high target:nontarget ratio. Positive localization of the radionuclide has been demonstrated in glioblastoma, astrocytoma, meningioma, and metastatic tumors. Labeled bleomycin appears superior to ^{99m}TcO$_4$ because of its affinity for tumors with high mitotic activity. It is more successful in demonstrating posterior fossa lesions due to its high target:nontarget ratio. Pertechnetate alone is still of value in demonstrating those tumors with an associated large blood volume or prolific neovascularity. Although ^{57}Co appears to be the label of choice for bleomycin, its high renal excretory rate (80% in 24 hours) necessitates urine collection and contamination problems. Another disadvantage is the delayed scanning interval, which appears to be 24 hours postinjection to obtain maximum tumor concentration of the radionuclide.

^{99m}Tc pertechnetate continues to be the agent of choice from the aspect of efficacy, availability, photon energy, radiation exposure to the patient, capabilities of current imaging devices, and cost.

Imaging Procedure

Normally, 10–15 mCi of pertechnetate is administered intravenously following preparation with 250–500 mg of potassium perchlorate to block uptake of the isotope by the choroid plexuses of the lateral and third ventricles, which may mimic tumor localization, and uptake by the thyroid gland. Previously, it had been demonstrated that perchlorate administration would not interfere with isotope localization in choroid plexus papillomas,[11] but a recent study suggests that this may not always be true.[12]

Scanning may be performed immediately following isotope administration, particularly in those tumors where the blood pool accounts for a larger portion of the abnormally increased uptake (i.e., highly vascular meningiomas, malignant melanomas, metastatic hypernephromas). Generally, a 30–60 minute interval is preferred to allow time for sufficient radionuclide to concentrate in the region of the tumor and to improve the target:nontarget ratio. A further delayed scan may be particularly beneficial in the diagnosis of intracerebral metastatic disease where a 3–4 hour interval may permit visualization of multiple lesions not present on earlier studies.

The general procedure employed in brain tumor localization is to obtain multiple projections since a suspected lesion should be visualized on at least two complementary views before the study is considered positive. Anterior, posterior, and both lateral views constitute the minimum study. A vertex view should be performed whenever parasagittal or intraventricular pathology is suspected or when a lesion is thought to extend across the midline. Whenever a vertex view is performed to visualize an anterior lesion it is advantageous to rinse the mouth with water prior to the study to remove residual background activity in the saliva.

Lesions located at the base of the brain or in the posterior fossa continue to present difficult diagnostic problems despite the use of tomographic scanners or a pinhole collimator. The use of atropine or increased perchlorate dosage may improve the quality of the scan by decreasing the degree of isotope localization in the mucous membranes and salivary glands. If a basilar or posterior fossa lesion is suspected but cannot be identified with $^{99m}TcO_4$, a second scan utilizing ^{197}Hg may aid in the delineation of pathology due to less interference from activity in adjacent soft tissues.

Interpretation

There are several routes of approach to the diagnosis of CNS tumors on the brain scan. Characteristically, tumors violate individual vessel regions and may extend across the midline. It is also unusual for tumors to undergo dramatic changes over a short period of time. A "doughnut" configuration with a central decrease in isotope concentration suggests necrotic, hemorrhagic, cystic, or degenerative changes. Adult lesions are more frequently supratentorial, while 66% of pediatric lesions tend to be infratentorial in location. Lesions less than 1.5–2.0 cm in size are usually not demonstrable and deep-seated lesions are best visualized by a rectilinear scanner with a focused collimator. Statistically, the most frequent brain tumors in descending order are: gliomas, metastatic lesions, and meningiomas.[13]

Temporal relationships are important. Usually scans are positive immediately following the onset of clinical symptomatology and isotope concentration increases and persists for a prolonged period of time. Thus, the longer the delay in performing the scan (i.e., 2–4 hours) the greater the likelihood that a study will be positive. A delayed

scan is of particular value in the diagnosis of intracranial metastatic disease because
there is a definite increase in the number of metastatic lesions visualized with time. The
amount of isotope accumulation also roughly parallels the malignant potential of the
lesion.

Geographic and radionuclidic distribution patterns contribute to the specific diagnosis of the type of lesion. Gliomas and glioblastoma multiforme (Fig. 1) are frequently
irregularly marginated and show patchy areas of decreased isotope distribution
representing regions of degeneration and necrosis as they enlarge and outgrow their
blood supply. There may be associated edema, and these tumors accumulate the isotope
in relation to time and malignant potential and have a tendency to cross the midline.
Glioblastoma multiforme presents almost exclusively in the cortical regions.

Metastatic lesions have a tendency toward multiplicity and increased isotope accumulation with time (Figs. 2a and 2b). They are usually circular with a more diffuse peripheral isotope distribution pattern due to circumferential edema. Following steroid
administration and/or radiation therapy there may be marked diminution in the size of
the lesion (Figs. 3a and 3c), often to the degree where localization would be difficult
without comparison to a previous study. Meningeal metastatic lesions present as peripheral plaques of increased isotope localization that may mimic vascular lesions (i.e.,
CVA, subdural hematoma).

Meningiomas (Figs. 4a, 4b, and 5) demonstrate early avid and homogeneous
concentration of radioactivity due to their abundant neovascularity. They are sharply

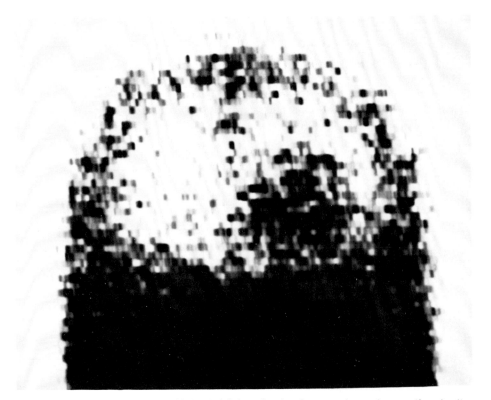

Fig. 1.   Large, irregularly marginated lesion in left frontal region demonstrating moderate uniform localization of ^{99m}Tc pertechnetate proven on biopsy to represent a glioblastoma multiforme.

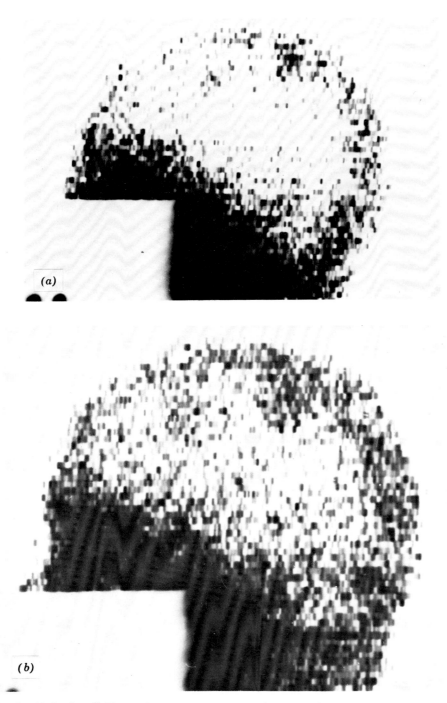

Fig. 2. (a) One-hour ^{99m}Tc pertechnetate scan revealing two focal areas of abnormal isotope localization in the left parietal region in a patient with known bronchogenic carcinoma. Left lateral view. (b) A 2½-hour delayed scan showing increased isotopic activity and better delineation of the metastatic brain lesions.

11

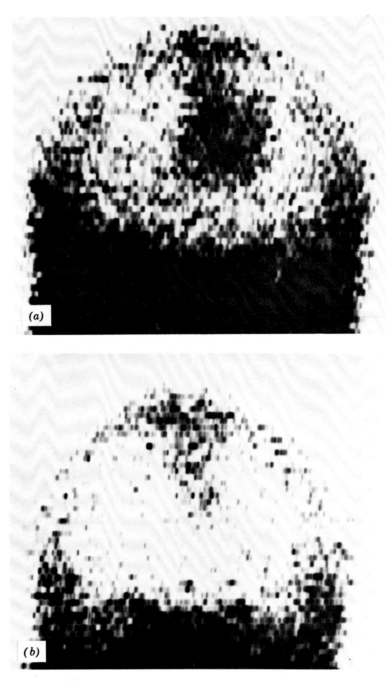

Fig. 3. (a) A large, abnormal area in the left frontal region demonstrated on a ^{99m}Tc pertechnetate brain scan in a patient with known bronchogenic carcinoma. (b) Marked diminution of isotope localization in the metastatic lesion following the administration of steroids. (c) Almost complete absence of isotope localization in the metastatic focus following radiation therapy.

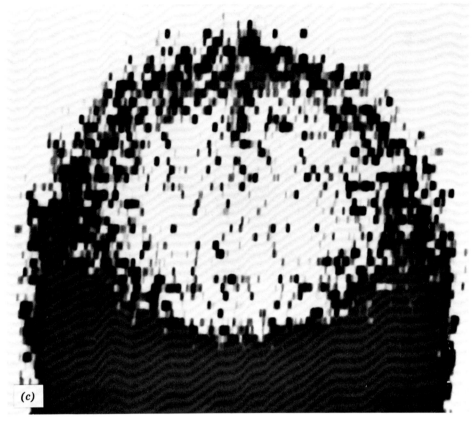

(c)

Fig. 3.   (Continued)

circumscribed and contiguous with the distribution of the arachnoid granulations on the meningeal surfaces. The most common locations are parasagittal, free-convexity, and sphenoid ridge.[14] Skull roentgenograms commonly demonstrate reactive sclerosis in the region of the tumor.

The most common posterior fossa tumors concentrating isotope are acoustic neuromas, cerebello-pontine angle tumors (Figs. 6a and 6b), and, in the pediatric patient, medulloblastomas and other gliomatous lesions. The tumor is usually located just lateral to the midline. Parasellar midline lesions include pituitary adenomas (Fig. 7), craniopharyngiomas (Fig. 8), and optic gliomas. Ependymomas and corpus callosum tumors are located at the level of the midbrain in the region of the ventricular system and have a propensity to cross the midline below the level of the sagittal sinus. Intraventricular tumors tend to assume the shape of the associated ventricles.

Diagnostic Accuracy

The diagnostic accuracy of any procedure must be considered within itself and in comparison with other diagnostic modalities. The three most common diagnostic approaches to neurologic tumors are the skull roentgenogram, the brain scan, and the arteriogram. The first two are benign, inoccuous procedures and can be considered for

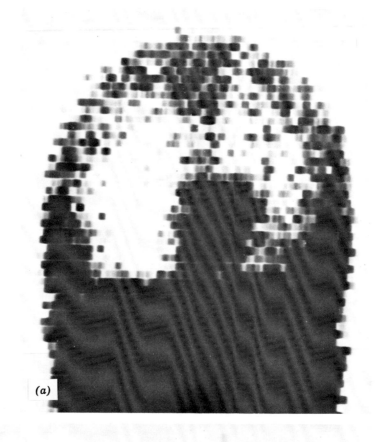

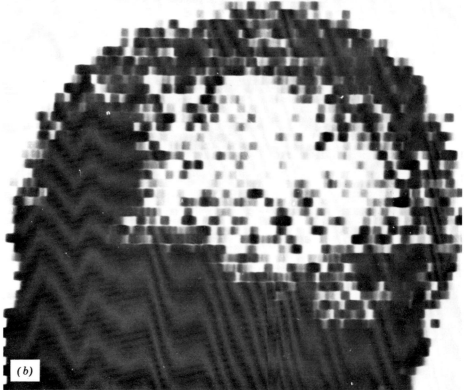

14

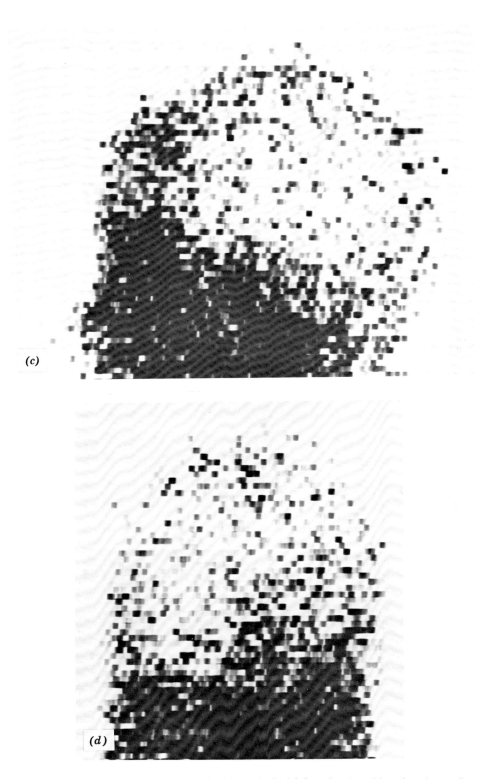

Fig. 4. (a and b) Large, well-circumscribed focal lesion in the left frontal region with uniform isotope distribution demonstrated on a ^{99m}Tc pertechnetate brain scan that was proven at surgery to represent an olfactory groove meningioma.

Fig. 4. (c and d) The olfactory groove meningioma again redemonstrated 72 hours following the administration of gallium-67 citrate.

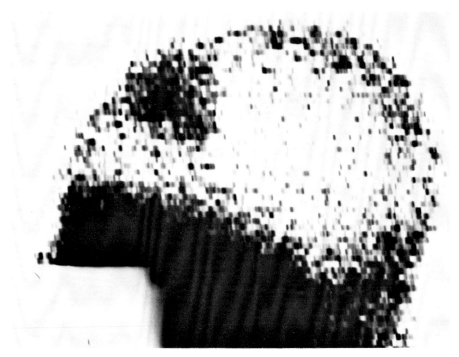

Fig. 5. ^{99m}Tc pertechnetate localized within a left parasagittal meningioma.

screening purposes. The arteriogram, however, is a somewhat more formidable procedure.

The comparative accuracy of these modalities is indicated in Table 1. This represents a compilation of data from two major investigators in separate institutions.[15, 16]

The plain skull roentgenogram has obviously limited usage but may be helpful when the lesion is calcified, as with meningiomas or craniopharyngiomas. If there is midline shift of a calcified pineal or if bone changes have occurred, this may be demonstrated. The arteriogram, on the other hand, may be more reliable than the brain scan in areas such as the sphenoid ridge. It is often less helpful, however, in lesions involving the occipital lobe, the posterior fossa, and the sellar region. It is also found to be less helpful in the presence of multiple small metastatic lesions.

The accuracy of brain scanning as it relates to specific tumors is indicated in Table 2.

TABLE 1   COMPARATIVE ACCURACY
OF NEURODIAGNOSTIC
PROCEDURES[15,16]

Method		
Skull x-ray	(80/208)	38%
Brain scan	(183/218)	84%
Arteriogram	(134/161)	83%

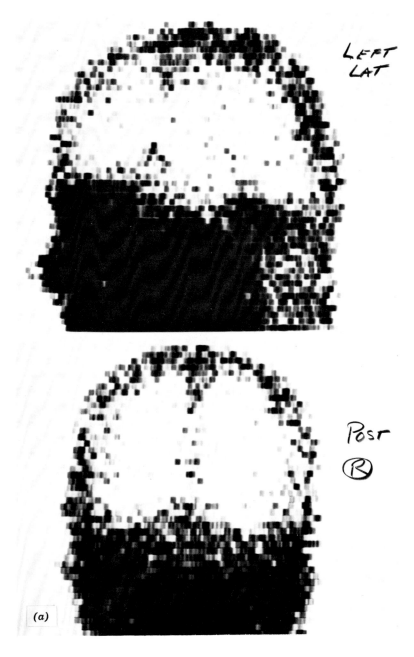

Fig. 6. (a) ^{99m}Tc pertechnetate localized within a left cerebello-pontine angle metastatic lesion. (b) Comparative right lateral view.

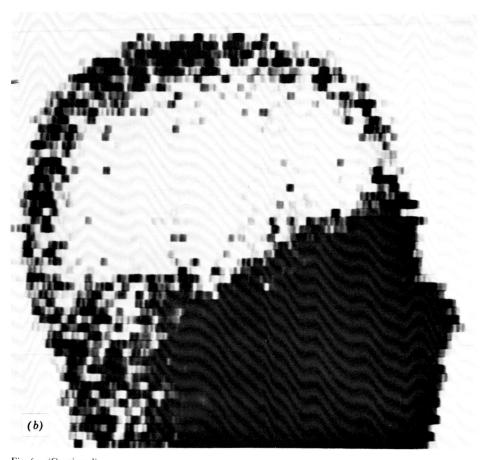

(b)

Fig. 6. (Continued)

TABLE 2 [17]   ACCURACY OF BRAIN
SCANNING IN SPECIFIC
TUMORS[a]

Tumor	Percent positive
Medulloblastoma	100
Glioblastoma	97
Meningioma	94
Metastases	93
Oligodendroglioma	83
Astrocytoma	76
Acoustic neurinoma	67
Pituitary	44
Ependymoma	33
[a] Total proven tumors	378
Correctly diagnosed	329 (87%)

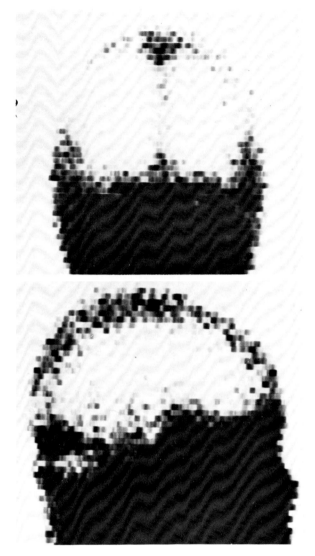

Fig. 7. Abnormal ^{99m}Tc pertechnetate localization in a midline lesion in the region of the sella turcica proven to represent a pituitary adenoma.

Based on the cell type suspected, this will aid in understanding the limitations of the procedure.

DYNAMIC FUNCTION STUDIES

Although static brain imaging can be performed with the rectilinear scanner as well as with the scintillation camera, the refinement and development of the camera with storage capability has fostered time-dependent studies in nuclear medicine.

Since the function of the brain is so critically dependent upon its blood supply, many techniques have been developed to assess the integrity of the cerebral circulation and to quantitate it.

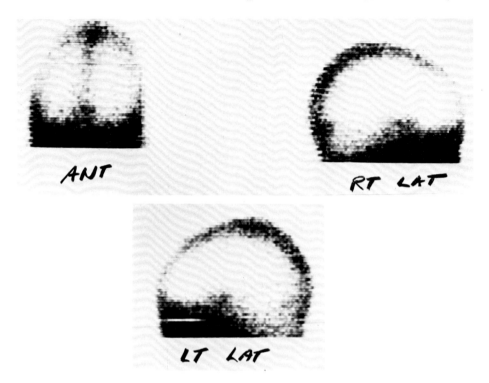

Fig. 8.   Abnormal localization of ^{99m}Tc pertechnetate within a midline lesion extending above the level of the sella turcica proven at surgery to represent a craniopharyngioma.

These began in 1948 with the report of a method using nitrous oxide by Kety and Schmidt.[18] Since that time, extensive application of diffusable and nondiffusable tracers has accompanied the use of external counters over various regions of the brain.[19] Because of their complexity, these methods have remained essentially in the research laboratory. With the increasing availability of the scintillation camera, interest in studying "cerebral blood flow" has grown rapidly.

The procedure consists of obtaining serial images of the brain following the intravenous injection of a bolus of a radionuclide. It is obvious that this procedure does not quantitate cerebral blood flow and is more analagous to radiographic cerebral angiography. Thus, various names have been applied: nuclear cerebral angiography, intravenous dynamic nucleography of the brain, and cerebral perfusion studies. The technique permits the comparative evaluation of hemispheric perfusion as well as comparative flow through the carotid arteries. Interpretation was originally performed by a visual inspection technique. With increasing sophistication of instrumentation it became possible to "flag" or denote certain "areas of interest" within the images obtained. Since the data have been stored on magnetic or video tape, a playback with electronically designated areas of interest permits the development of activity histograms in the form of an analog display of the digital data.

The diagnostic value of this procedure becomes apparent when we consider that most conventional static brain scans do not clearly distinguish between neoplasms and vascular problems such as cerebral vascular accidents and arteriovenous malformations. The diagnosis was previously based on the clinical impression and on the appearance of the radiographic contrast angiogram. The angiogram is not always desirable because of its patient morbidity and untoward pharmacologic effects.

Technique

The patient is positioned beneath the detector of the scintillation camera, and the projection utilized is quite variable. Most often the studies are done with the patient in either the anterior or posterior projection, although lateral, vertex, and fronto vertex views have been reported by various authors.[20, 21] An intravenous injection of a bolus of ^{99m}Tc pertechnetate in a dosage range of 10–20 mCi is administered through the antecubital fossa.

Serial images are then collected by the scintillation camera with accumulation intervals of 0.5–3.0 seconds, depending upon the instrumentation. The data is stored most commonly on magnetic tape. The playback of the collected images demonstrates the flow of the radionuclide through the internal and external carotid arteries and occasionally the vertebral artery. Perfusion of the brain is visualized and both the arterial and venous phases are recorded (Fig. 9).

Areas of interest are identified electronically: the cerebral hemispheres and areas over the carotid arteries. Data from the subsequent playback of the tape with the areas of interest flagged is treated in several ways. The information can be fed through a

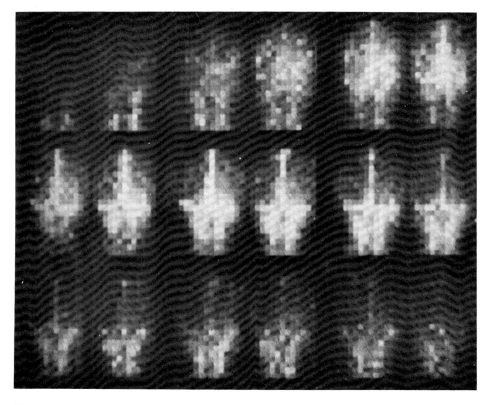

Fig. 9. Serial images demonstrating flow of ^{99m}Tc bolus through the carotid arteries and perfusion of the hemisphere with both arterial and venous phase, posterior projection.

strip-chart recorder and the analog curves created as in Fig. 10. In newer instrumentation these curves are created by an on-line computer and the histogram is
displayed on a television monitor readout (Fig. 11). This permits us to detect asym-
metry of the carotid flow and hemispheric perfusion and to effectively quantitate that
difference. Figure 12 demonstrates a study with the cerebral perfusion curve reaching a
maximum peak approximately 16% lower than the contralateral side. This patient had
suffered a cerebral vascular accident. The static brain scan revealed a well-defined
concentration of the radioisotope, suggesting an intracranial lesion.

Interpretation

Several characteristic perfusion patterns have been developed.[21, 22] In a patient with a
positive localization on static brain scanning, evaluation of the initial perfusion as well
as the washout phase may reveal: (1) increased perfusion over the lesion that maintains
during washout or (2) normal perfusion over the lesion which initially develops a positive

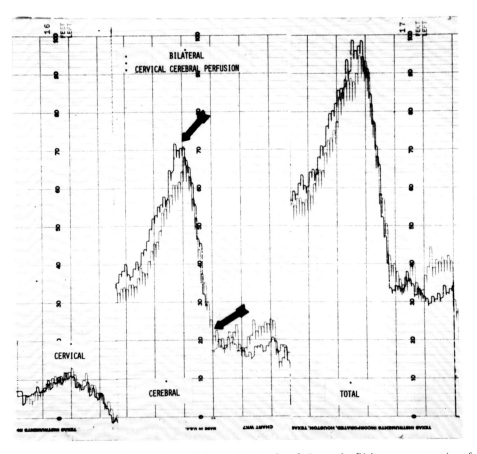

Fig. 10.   Analog curves of a normal carotid flow and cerebral perfusion study. Right curve: summation of
flow through both carotids and hemispheres; middle curves: comparative hemispheric perfusion; left curves:
comparative carotid blood flow.

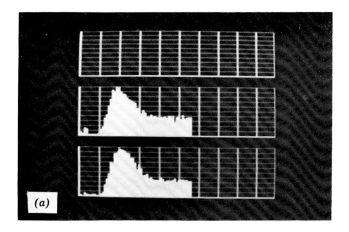

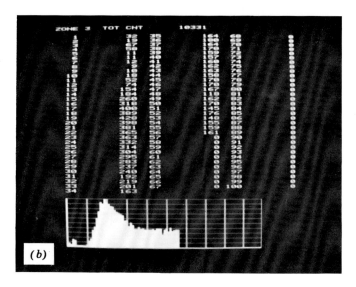

Fig. 11. (a) Computer-generated activity histogram representing bilateral cerebral hemispheric perfusion. (b) Histogram with digital data for 100-point curve.

target:background ratio during the washout phase. Both these patterns represent primary or secondary neoplasm. Increased perfusion demonstrated over the lesion initially but disappearing during the washout phase represents arteriovenous malformation. Initial decreased perfusion that later develops a positive static finding is characteristic of vascular lesions such as intracerebral hematoma, vascular occlusive disease, and subdural hematoma.

In a patient suspected of an intracerebral lesion, we suggest that brain scanning be performed initially. If a positive lesion is identified on the brain scan, then the radionuclide cerebral angiogram should be used as an adjunct. The data concerning the carotid blood flow and cerebral perfusion to the region of the identified lesion can be extremely helpful in making a more accurate differential diagnosis of the pathological process.

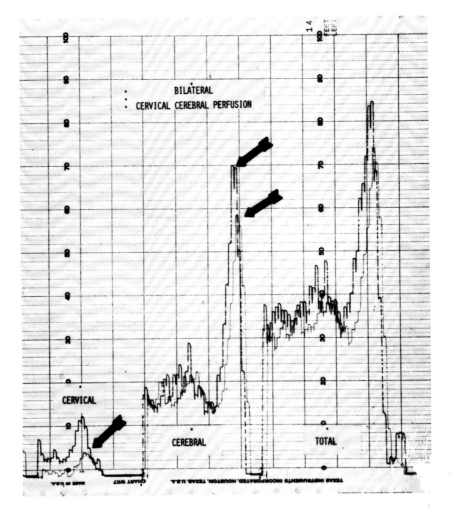

Fig. 12.   Analog curves demonstrating asymmetrical cerebral perfusion and asymmetrical carotid blood flow in a patient with a cerebrovascular accident.

EVALUATION OF CEREBROSPINAL FLUID DYNAMICS

Although neurophysiologists have been aware for many years that many pathologic conditions cause serious alterations in the normal cerebrospinal fluid kinetics, a full understanding of the production and resorption of CSF has not been obtained. Likewise, there has not been a relatively simple technique for studying the patient with suspected abnormalities, particularly tumor involvement.

Originally, various organic dyes were injected directly into the ventricular system and their distribution in the CSF spaces was noted.[23] The first radionuclide used was [198]Au which was injected into the lumbar arachnoid space in animals.[24] The availability of high-specific-activity ^{131}I-labeled human serum albumin made possible a number of studies and techniques utilizing nuclear imaging equipment.[25] The terms "radioisotope cisternography" and "radioisotope myelography" refer to the technique where the radionuclide is injected intrathecally and the term "radioisotope ventriculography" is used to describe those studies where the radionuclide is administered intraventricularly.

Over the past several years radioisotope cisternography has slowly evolved from a research tool to an important diagnostic modality for the clinical evaluation of pathology involving the cerebrospinal fluid circulatory system.

CSF Circulation

CSF is almost entirely produced within the ventricular system from a dual source at a rate related to the surface area of the choroid plexus and ventricular wall. The choroid plexus produces cerebrospinal fluid by active secretion.[26] The principle source of protein (i.e., albumin) appears to be the plasma, entering the cerebrospinal fluid both from the choroid plexus and intact arachnoid. Because protein generates significant osmotic pressure, its reabsorption will obligate water, creating a "bulk flow" of cerebrospinal fluid from site of origin to sites of reabsorption. The greatest reabsorption of protein is normally through the parasagittal or Pacchionian granulations.

Milhorat[27] describes the bulk flow circulatory pathway as follows: CSF that is formed in the lateral ventricles passes out through the paired interventricular foramina of Monroe to reach the third ventricle. The fluid then flows caudally through the Aquaduct of Sylvius and fourth ventricle, where it passes into the subarachnoid space by one of three exits: two lateral Foramina of Luschka, which direct fluid around the brain stem into the cerebellopontine and prepontine cisterns, and a midline Foramen of Magendie, which directs fluid through the vallecula into the cisterna magna. From the cisterna magna, fluid passes in several directions: (1) superiorly into the subarachnoid space investing the cerebellar hemispheres, (2) caudally into the spinal subarachnoid space. and (3) cephalad into the basilar cisterns. From the basilar cisterns the bulk flow of fluid continues along two major routes: (1) ventrally through the interpenduncular and prechiasmatic cisterns passing mainly through the Sylvian fissure and callosal cisterns to the subarachnoid space investing the lateral and frontal aspects of the cerebral hemispheres and (2) dorsomedially through the ambient cisterns and cisterna vena magna cerebri from which fluid passes to the subarachnoid space investing the medial and posterior aspects of the cerebral hemispheres. The circulation through the subarachnoid space presumably terminates at the level of the dural sinuses where absorption occurs across the arachnoid villi. The hydrostatic pressure and dural sinus pressure differential acts as a "suction pump" contributing to cephalic movement.

a radionuclide injected into the cerebrospinal fluid via the lumbar space will ascend to the level of the cisterna magna and basilar cisterns to eral circulatory pathway. Since the bulk flow of fluid is passing out of the lar system, the hydrostatic pressure is sufficient to prevent intraventricular localization.

Radiopharmaceuticals

Although the most widely used radionuclide has been ^{131}I-human serum albumin, others must be considered. The current radiopharmaceuticals of choice for radioisotope cisternography include:

[131]I-human serum albumin (HSA)

[99m]Tc-human serum albumin (HSA)

[169]Yb-diethylenetriamine pentaacetic acid (DTPA)

[111]In-transferrin

[111]In-diethylenetriamine pentaacetic acid (DTPA)

Each radionuclide employed has advantages and disadvantages and the final choice is predicated on the nature of the clinical problem.

^{99m}Tc-HSA with its short half-life, low gamma energy, and high photon flux is best suited for camera studies of patients in the pediatric age group. Both ^{131}I-HSA and [169]Yb-DTPA deliver a relatively high radiation dose to the spinal cord. In addition, [169]Yb-DTPA, following absorption from the cerebrospinal fluid, equilibrates with the extracellular fluid and is removed from the blood by means of glomerular filtration with 90% renal excretion in 24 hours. Consequently, the use of [169]Yb-DTPA is precluded in the presence of renal insufficiency.[28] ^{131}I-HSA with its low photon flux and relatively higher gamma energy is best imaged with the rectilinear scanner. [111]In and [169]Yb have a lower energy and a higher photon flux, permitting adequate imaging with camera systems.

Finally, both ^{131}I-HSA and ^{111}In-DTPA have been reported[29, 30] to cause the sequelae of aseptic meningitis secondary to the amount of protein or carrier present.

Technique

The major route of isotope administration is via the lumbar subarachnoid space utilizing standard sterile lumbar puncture techniques. Generally, the radionuclide is mixed with a small volume (1–2 ml) of cerebrospinal fluid prior to injection. Manometric measurements, excessive barbotage, and manipulation should be avoided. In the past it had been thought that prior recent lumbar punctures or pneumoencephalography would negate the study by interfering with isotope flow or permitting leakage of the radiopharmaceutical from the dural sac. However, recent studies[31] indicate that the technique of radionuclide administration is the most crucial factor. Although delay may improve the incidence of success, a subarachnoid injection usually assures an adequate study.

Postinjection, a straight column of activity is normally seen in a midline location with small dural sleeves present at intervals along the longitudinal extent (Fig. 13). At 1 hour the radionuclide should enter the cisterna magna and 3 hours postinjection the initial scan is performed. At this time, there should be definite activity seen within the suprasellar, callosal, and quadrigeminal cisterns and along the Sylvian fissures (Fig. 14). If there is no evidence of isotope activity above the level of the cisterna magna at the 3-hour interval and there is no clinical suspicion of the presence of a block, a scan of the thoraco-lumbar region should be obtained. This usually will demonstrate a pattern indicative of faulty technique with resultant misdirection of the radionuclide.

DiChiro et al[32] describe several patterns:

1. A broad diffuse pattern of spinal activity with a central columnar void (representing the subarachnoid space) and "christmas tree" pattern of delicate branching extensions of activity indicating an epidural injection. The column stops at the atlanto-occipital joint at the point of termination of the epidural space.

2. A "railroad track" pattern consisting of a double band of activity surrounding the negative defect of the subarachnoid space of the *cul-de-sac* indicating a subdural injection (Fig. 15).

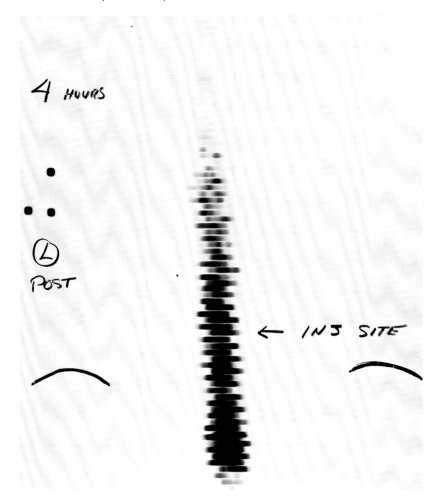

Fig. 13. Normal pattern of isotope distribution within the lumbar subarachnoid space.

3. A midline or central pattern that may persist for 48 hours indicating a spinal ligament or muscle injection.

4. A combination of the above may occur.

Imaging is then performed 24 and 48 hours postinjection. At 24 hours the radionuclide extends over the convexity and by 48 hours (Fig. 16) it is primarily localized to the parasagittal region with a decreased count rate indicative of partial absorption. In children cerebrospinal fluid hydrodynamics are more rapid so that this radionuclide distribution pattern is normally present at the 12–24 hour interval.

Pathophysiology

Although radioisotope cisternography has been employed primarily for the evaluation of hydrocephalus, it is capable of detecting the presence of tumor and offering a differential diagnosis based on the anatomic location of the alteration in cerebrospinal fluid and flow.

Tumors are a rare cause of *communicating* (Figs. 17 and 18) hydrocephalus, although this has been known to occur when protein reabsorption is blocked by tumor presenting in a parasagittal location, or secondary to chronic inflammatory changes produced by diffuse leptomeningeal tumors:

1.   Primary tumors (i.e., sarcoma).
2.   Secondary tumors (i.e., metastatic carcinoma, lymphoma).
3.   CNS tumor seeding CSF pathways (i.e., glioblastoma, medulloblastoma, choroid plexus papilloma).

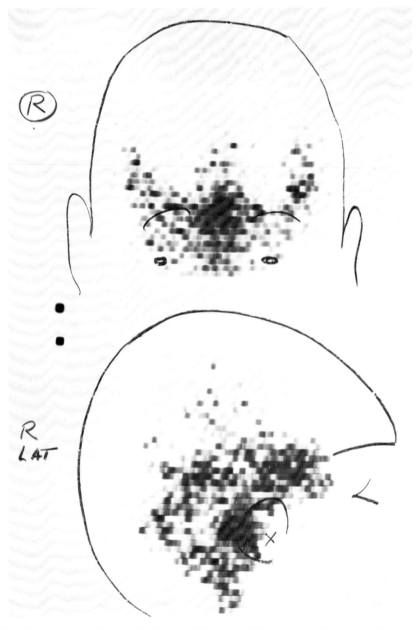

Fig. 14.   Normal pattern of isotope distribution within the basal cisterns at the 3-hour interval.

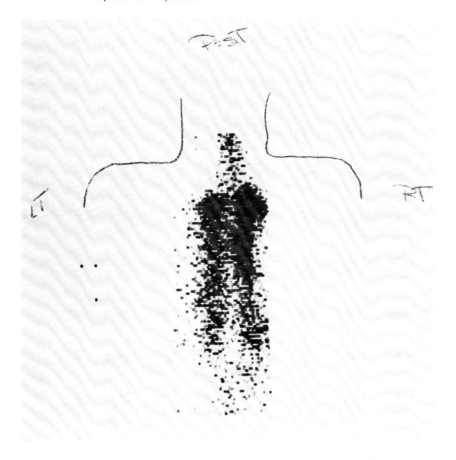

Fig. 15. "Railroad track" pattern suggesting subdural isotope administration. The central linear area of lucency represents the spinal cord.

Milhorat[27] acknowledges that tumors are the most common cause of acquired *noncommunicating* hydrocephalus (Fig. 19). This condition presents by cisternography as a block to the flow of radionuclide at the level of the basal cisterns and Sylvian fissures due to ventricular expansion with subsequent cerebrospinal fluid pathway compression. Radioisotope ventriculography, either by direct injection or administered via the reservoir of a ventricular shunt, may outline the tumor mass or demonstrate the anatomic site of obstruction.

The lateral ventricles may be selectively obstructed by tumors arising within these cavities. The most common intraventricular tumors include choroid plexus papillomas, ependymomas, tubers, infiltrating gliomas, metastatic tumors, and meningiomas. Any large hemispheral mass may obstruct the foramen of Monroe of the opposite lateral ventricle and produce contralateral hydrocephalus. The third ventricle may be obstructed inferiorly by parenchymal or extraaxial tumors and posteriorly by pineal tumors. The Aqueduct of Sylvius is a frequent site of obstruction by tumor due to its considerable length and relatively narrow caliber. In the vast majority of cases, the tumors responsible lie outside the brain stem. The primary mechanism of obstruction is

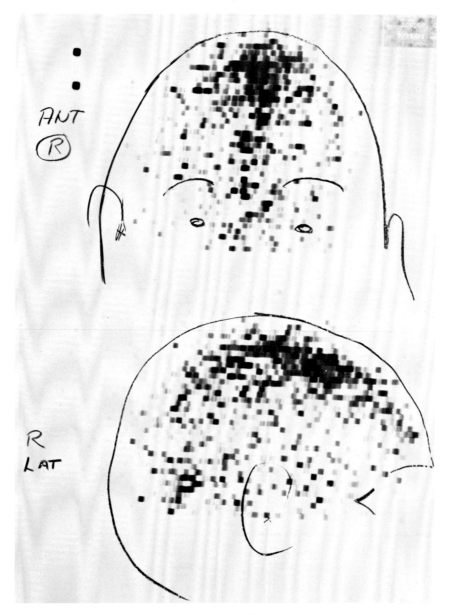

Fig. 16.   Normal parasagittal distribution of isotope 48 hours postinjection.

by "kinking" and/or angulation. Generally, masses in the posterior fossa are most likely to cause hydrocephalus.

A recent study by Mamo et al[33] establishes the importance of radioisotope cisternography in the diagnosis of cerebellopontine angle tumors. This technique permits "physiological" visualization of the periencephalic cisterns and "may confirm the existence of tumor where conventional methods give only negative or doubtful results."

On the posterior view a filling defect may be present on the side of the tumor with unilateral deformity and encroachment on the cerebellopontine and prepontine cisterns.

Internal and superior extension of the tumor causes deformity and amputation of the preaxial cisterns, while inferior extension causes deformity and amputation of the lateral aspect of the cisterna magna. In the lateral projection, partial amputation of the superior portion of the cisternal image is seen. Attention should be paid to cisternal anatomy for the diagnosis of lesions that are in locations conducive to alterations in the cerebrospinal fluid spaces.

Ommaya et al[34] have presented a classification of nontraumatic cerebrospinal fluid

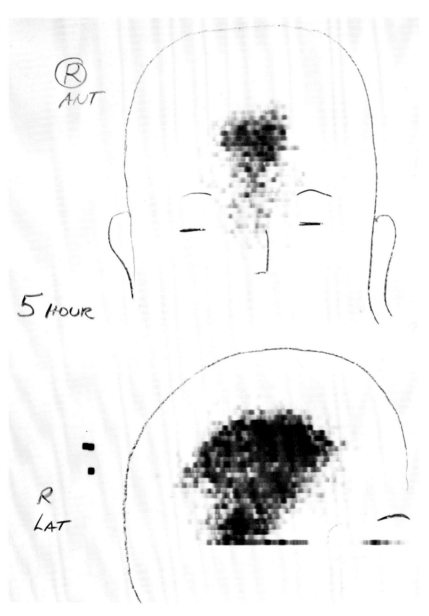

Fig. 17.   Pattern of isotope distribution in communicating hydrocephalus with isotope in an intraventricular location at the 5-hour interval persisting through 48 hours.

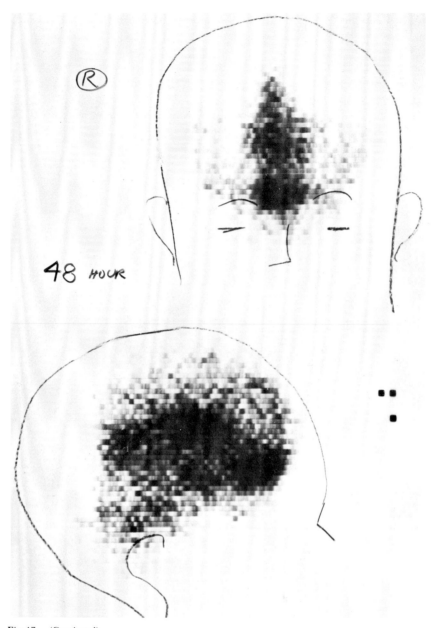

Fig. 17. (Continued)

rhinorrhea, in terms of the mechanism of leakage, into two categories: "high pressure" and "normal pressure." In the high-pressure category the leakage of cerebrospinal fluid usually acts as a safety valve. Closure of the valve will invariably worsen the patient's condition if the causative lesion is not treated. More than one-half of the patients with nontraumatic rhinorrhea were high-pressure leaks and were due to tumors. In their series 40% were pituitary tumors, closely followed by acoustic neurinomas (20%) and cerebellar gliomas (20%). Although pituitary tumors are the lesions most commonly causing rhinorrhea, it should be noted that CSF rhinorrhea is a rare complication of such tumors. The fistulas may be created in two ways, either directly by erosion of meninges and bone, or indirectly via pressure erosion of anatomically fragile areas of the skull base (frequently at the level of the cribriform plate).

Thus, a combination of accurate radiographic studies and radioisotope cisternography will yield the best diagnostic results. In the series, cisternography gave the final diagnostic answer in all the cases in which it was employed. The fissure site was denoted either by scan delineation of an abnormal collection or track of radionuclide, or by the appropriate placement and subsequent well counting of nasal pledgets.

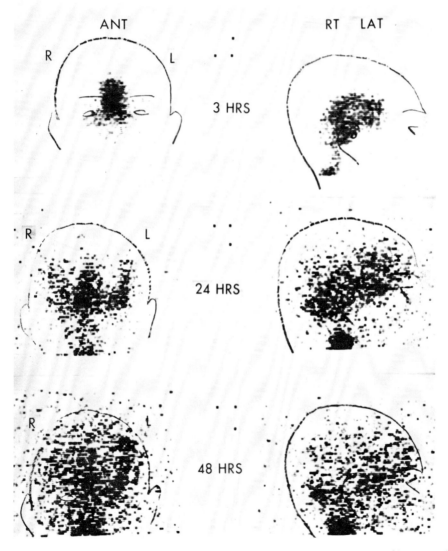

Fig. 18.   Another example of communicating hydrocephalus with apparent disappearance of isotope at the 24-hour interval suggesting "compensated" form. Note: A residual collection of isotope just below the level of the cisterna magna which represents a partial epidural injection.

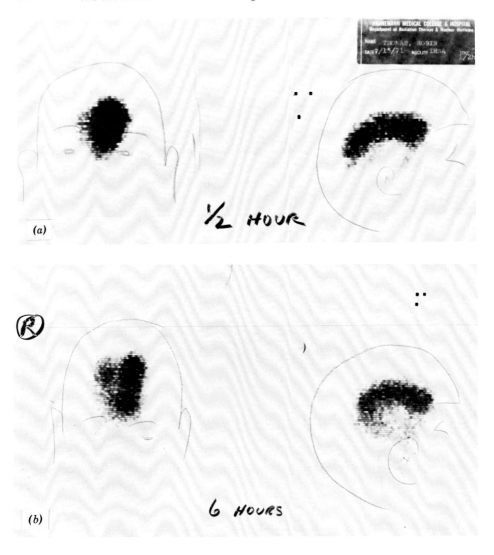

Fig. 19. A typical isotope ventriculogram demonstrating the usual isotope distribution pattern in the presence of noncommunicating hydrocephalus. Note: The delayed visualization of the right ventricle with time and failure of the isotope to descend below the level of the third ventricle.

MYELOSCINTIGRAPHY

Myeloscintigraphy or radionuclide myelography is an accurate, reliable and safe method of localizing obstruction caused by mass lesions in the spinal canal. This procedure originated with Bauer and Yuhl in 1953.[35] In their initial studies they injected 100 μCi of ^{131}I-sodium iodide intrathecally into normal rabbits and into rabbits with surgically induced spinal blocks. While these studies were very successful in localizing the level of the block, the radionuclide was rapidly cleared from the subarachnoid space. This would not allow for delayed examinations or additional views. These investigators then chose to substitute ^{131}I-human serum albumin (^{131}I-

HSA) as their tracer agent, affording a slower diffusion and absorption rate. In addition to ^{131}I-HSA, ^{99m}Tc-HSA, ^{111}In-transferrin, ^{111}In-DTPA, and ^{169}Yb-DTPA[37] may also be used as in cisternography.

Technique

The patient is prepared and draped in the normal lumbar puncture position. A spinal tap is performed and 1–2 ml of spinal fluid is removed. ^{131}I-HSA in dosage of 100 μCi and high specific activity is injected and this is followed by the previously withdrawn CSF. In an effort to decrease the side effects, 100 mg of hydrocortisone can be given the night preceding and 1 hour preceding the intrathecal injection. The maximum amount of albumin injected should not exceed 4 mg. The patient is normally scanned in the prone position from 15 minutes to several hours postinjection. With both ^{131}I-HSA and ^{99m}Tc-HSA some radionuclide will dissociate from the albumin and be localized in the thyroid gland. To protect the gland, Lugol's solution or potassium perchlorate should be given prior to injection of the radionuclide.

In a normal myeloscintigram there is uniform radionuclide localization throughout the entire subarachnoid space to the level of the cisterna magnum in 1–2 hours. In the event that the radionuclide is injected in the epidural space rather than in the subarachnoid space, the tracer ascends through the epidural space to the level of the foramen magnum where it disappears. As noted previously, this pattern is called "railroad tracking" and can be likened to radionuclide around the periphery of an elongated cylinder. In the event there is an obstruction to the flow of CSF, there will be an area of increased radionuclide localization with activity absent superiorly. If the block is only partial, the concentration will be decreased, rather than absent. An advantage of the myeloscintigram is that the study may be repeated relatively soon without interference from the previous examination. Voutilainen et al[36] performed myeloscintigraphy on 22 patients, with 17 positive studies. Seven patients were found to have primary tumors, while 8 patients proved to have metastatic lesions. The other two positive cases were due to disc disease.

RADIONUCLIDE LOCALIZATION OF INTRAOCULAR AND INTRAORBITAL TUMORS

The use of radioisotopes in ophthalmology centers around the use of radiophosphorous (^{32}P) for the diagnosis of uveal melanomas. Although the study has been in existence for over 20 years it has recently been refined to include the examination and detection of small lesions suspected of being melanomas.

Melanomas constitute a majority of malignant intraocular tumors. The ability to exclude or include them in differential diagnosis is of major importance to the ophthalmologist. Many lesions may simulate melanomas and since enucleation of an otherwise healthy eye could result from a false positive diagnosis of melanoma, the diagnostic technique must be accurate. A study by Shields and Zimmerman from specimens submitted to the Armed Forces Institute of Pathology[40] revealed that a 20% error in the clinical diagnosis of malignant melanoma may be the national average. More recent studies have shown that in teaching institutions, such as the Wills Hospital, the average misdiagnosis drops dramatically when consultation and corroborative clinical testing are

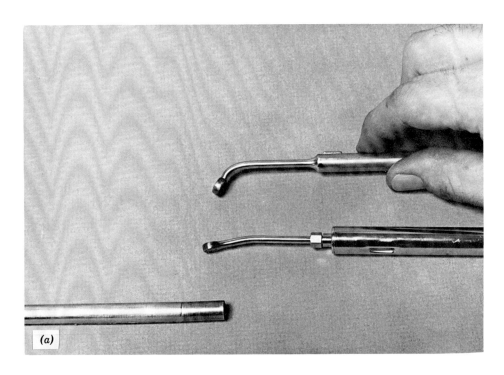

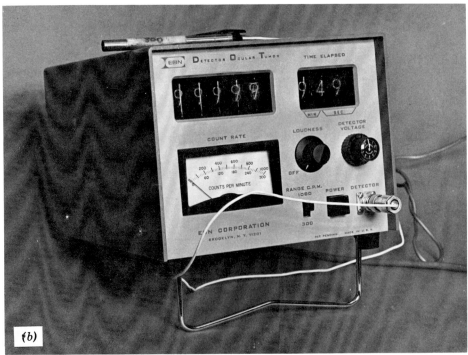

Fig. 20. (a) Geiger-Mueller detectors for ^{32}P-uptake studies. (b) Ratemeter system for ocular probes.

36

employed.[41] Several tests are available for the diagnosis of melanomas. These consist of transillumination, fluorescein angiography, indirect ophthalmoscopy, ultrasound, and the ^{32}P test. The use of all these techniques, as well as consultation among experienced retinal surgeons, can reduce the error in diagnosis to about 2%.

The ^{32}P test was first reported in the ophthalmic literature in 1950 by Thomas et al.[42] At that time the test was limited to anterior accessible lesions utilizing a specially designed Geiger-Mueller probe. The detector unit consisted of the probe attached to a simple ratemeter that displayed counts arising from the lesion. The opposite eye was used as a control, and counts were taken from all four quadrants. A fundamental limitation consisted of an inability to place a detector on lesions situated posterior to the equatorial plane of the globe. Several investigators developed specially designed probes for this purpose[43] (Figs. 20a and 20b). Unfortunately, detection with these probes was unsatisfactory because of an inability to accurately localize the position of the probe over the posterior lesion with the direct ophthalmoscope. Because of this serious limitation the technique was not used for over a decade.

Simultaneously, great strides were being made in retinal surgery with the development of the indirect ophthalmoscope and surgical techniques involving precise localization of posterior retinal tears. It was a simple step for Hagler, Jarrett, and Humphrey[44] in 1969 to apply these localization techniques in conjunction with the previously designed posterior probe. The study was instantly resurrected at several centers as an adjunct in diagnosis of uveal melanomas.[45] Statistics from these centers continue to demonstrate that the accuracy of the test in eyes with confirmed histologic specimens is 95%.

Radiopharmaceuticals

The radionuclide used is the 14.3 day half-life, pure beta-emitter ^{32}P, as sodium phosphate. The maximum energy is 1.71 MeV and the average energy is 695 keV. The amount of ^{32}P incorporated within tissue is determined by measuring the total number of beta particles reaching the surface where the detector is located. The beta particles measured come from a definite volume of tissue. The limits of the measurement are determined by tissue-detector geometry, the maximum energy of ^{32}P, and the tissue density. With measurements of radiation at the surface of the tissue, these factors became more important. The variables include the existence of a third dimension and the addition of biological factors such as the heterogeneous nature of tissues and the dynamic processes that are occurring within living tissues.

Absorption of the beta particles is the most important factor in tissue-surface measurements. Absorption curves obtained by measuring the transmission through different thicknesses of absorbers are complicated by scattering phenomena and the heterogeneous energy distribution of the particles. In tissue-surface measurements the absorption is still more difficult to evaluate. To approximate tissue penetration the mass attenuation coefficient of water may be used to characterize tissue penetration. It has been demonstrated that beta particles will penetrate an average of 4 mm of tissue. The placement of the probe over the area of the lesion must be very accurate (at least within 1 or 2 mm), otherwise the counts decrease dramatically and a false negative test may result.[46]

Technique

Seven hundred microcuries of ^{32}P is injected intravenously. If the lesion is located anterior to the equator and is accessible to the "anterior" probe, counts are made at 1, 24, and 48 hours. The criterion for a positive test is activity greater than 30% in the first hour increasing in 48 hours over the normal eye. If the lesion is located posterior to the equator of the globe, the posterior probe is utilized. An injection of 700 μCi of ^{32}P is given 48 hours prior to the measurement. The study can be done under local or general anesthesia depending on whether or not enucleation of the globe is intended. The lesion is accurately localized with the indirect ophthalmoscope and its margins marked with diathermy on the sclera. The probe is then placed directly over the lesion and counts are recorded (Fig. 21). The opposite quadrant of the same eye is used as a control. A positive test utilizes the criterion of Goldberg and Kara and co-workers[47] who found that most positive lesions in their study showed a differential of counts 60% greater than the normal eye 48 hours after injection. The use of this criterion has continued to yield results which support those of other investigators.

The theoretical basis for the application of radiophosphorous as a diagnostic agent resides in the work of Thomas et al[48] who have shown that phosphorous accumulates in the RNA, DNA acid, and phospholipid fractions of tumors. These studies have supported the clinical finding that tumors continue to localize ^{32}P in greater concentration than normal or inflammatory lesions for periods of 2–5 days.

It has been suggested by Holst[45] that if the concentration of ^{32}P in the uvea and vitreous gel surrounding the tumor demonstrates a standard proportionality then it is possible that all lesions greater than 3 mm in size should give a positive ^{32}P test. Packer and Lange[49] showed that there is no relationship between uptake and tumor size; only ^{32}P concentration affects uptake. Although this would lead some to believe that there exists a definite relationship between tumor cell type and percent uptake, we have not been able to support this concept. This fact would tend to further invalidate the specificity of this clinical test, since it is also well known that ^{32}P does not concentrate solely in melanomas. Fortunately, melanomas are the most common of malignant uveal tumors and most of the lesions seen clinically are larger than 3 mm.

With the increase in the sophistication of diagnostic techniques it has now become possible for the clinician to identify lesions smaller than 3 mm in the ocular fundus as possible malignant melanomas. Recently, the introduction of a semiconductor detector[50] seems to offer a more sensitive detection system than the Geiger-Mueller tube for smaller lesions.

Recently, work with noncontact methods for the detection of intraocular melanomas has received closer attention. These tests center on the specificity of concentration of chloroquine[51] in uveal tissue. One technique uses ^{125}I-labeled chloroquine. At first a modified 5-in. NaI (Tl) crystal was used as a detector. Later, the same authors reported the use of a specially designed hand-held scintillation probe.

Although the series of patients studied was small, simplicity of the method would tend to outweigh the more elaborate technique of the ^{32}P test. Despite the fact that the test is specific for pigmented melanomas, it is possible that false negative findings may result with amelanotic lesions. The problem of the number of excess counts in the affected eye over background and what constitutes normal differences between two eyes has yet to be settled. The use of ^{123}I-chloroquine in similar situations has been reported by other authors.[52]

Verin et al[53] have utilized the scintillation camera and a pinhole collimator along with ^{131}I-diiodofluorescein and ^{131}I-chloroquine in separate doses. With this method they state that a positive dioiodfluorescein test (20% difference in counts) and a positive chloroquine test may also indicate malignancy. A positive diiodofluorescein and negative chloroquine test signifies a vascular lesion, retinoblastoma, or metastatic malignancy.

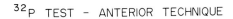

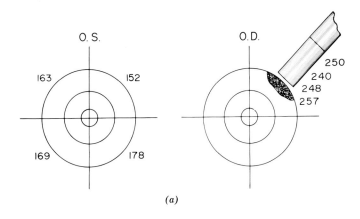

(a)

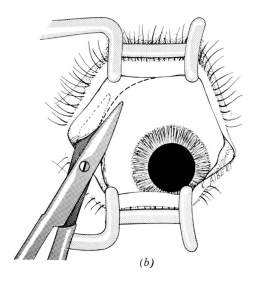

(b)

Fig. 21. (a) Probe counting technique (O.S. is control eye). (b) Incision of conjunctiva for insertion of probe. (c) Localization of tumor with diathermy marks and indirect ophthalmoscopy. (d) Position of posterior probe over diathermy marks for counting.

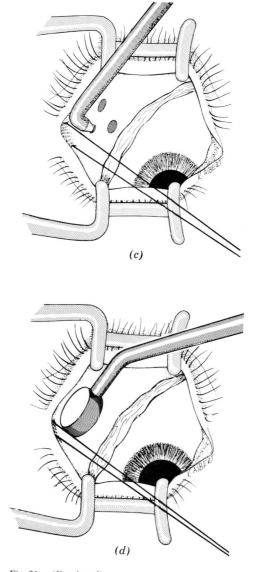

(c)

(d)

Fig. 21.   (Continued)

[83]Rb and ^{86}Rb were used by Leopold and co-workers[54] in 1964 in an effort to localize intraocular tumors, but their experiences with these isotopes were unrewarding. [67]Ga has also been used clinically in an attempt to localize intraocular tumors. Although positive images were found in two cases of ciliary body melanomas by Brady, Croll, Carmichael, and Wallner,[55] Heuer, Ehlers, and Hansen[56] have not found the test of value for localization of tumors on a quantitative or imaging basis.

Cappin and Greaves[57] have used [197]Hg-chlormerodrin as a diagnostic agent for ocular tumors with a 79.2% success rate. [203]Hg gammaencephalography has been employed by Fillipone and co-workers[58] in diagnosis of cerebral and intraocular tumors. Hopping[59] also reported on the use of this agent, but discontinued it in favor of [197]Hg because of its lower radiation dose to the patient.

The differential diagnosis of unilateral exophthalmos must always include the possibility of orbital malignancy. Meningiomas, hemangiomas, optic nerve gliomas, hamartomas, and sarcomas can be localized with radionuclide imaging[60-63] [197]Hg-chlormerodrin and ^{99m}Tc pertechnetate are the two isotopes commonly used to detect possible intraorbital lesions. Rectilinear scanning or imaging techniques with *en face*, modified Waters and lateral projections are used. One millicurie of radiotechnetium or 1.5 mCi of [197]Hg-chlormerodrin is injected intravenously 2–3 hours prior to scanning with either agent. It is well to precede the [197]Hg test with a renal blocking agent such as melluride and the radiotechnetium test with potassium perchlorate and atropine to remove interference from sinus walls and glandular areas surrounding the orbital cavities (Fig. 22). The standard imaging procedures should be accompanied by orbital and skull x-rays. The studies are complimentary and it has been noted that if both the isotope and radiographic studies are positive for an orbital mass, the evidence is overwhelming for malignancy or pseudotumor.

A malignant orbital mass will usually present as a focal area of isotope concentration within the orbital area (Figs. 23 and 24). Inflammatory lesions are usually diffuse in character and demonstrate irregular areas of activity. It is not common for thyroid

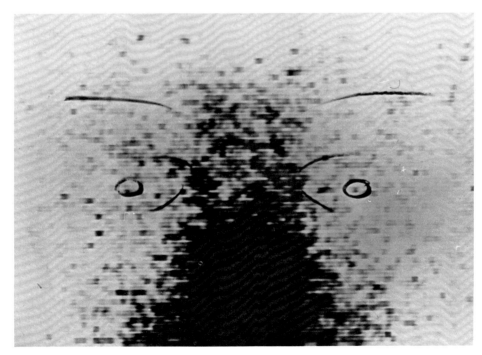

Fig. 22. Normal orbital scan.

exophthalmos to demonstrate increased isotope uptake within the orbital tissues and if it does is a rather irregular diffuse localization of isotope similar to that seen with inflammatory lesions. Thyroid function studies are often useful in ruling out this problem. Radionuclide arteriography can also be used to help rule out vascular lesions and arteriovenous communications.

The postoperative course of all surgically extirpated orbital masses can be followed on a regular basis with radionuclide studies. It is possible to detect minimal recurrences of a tumor when serial scanning is performed at regular intervals.

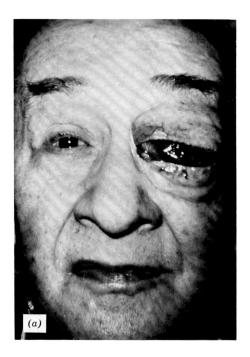

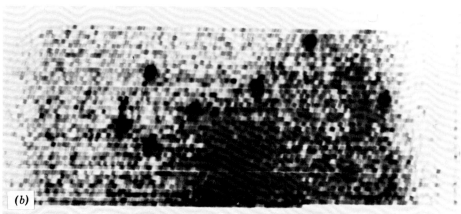

Fig. 23.   (a) Patient with sphenoid ridge meningioma. (b) Orbital scan showing localization left orbit.

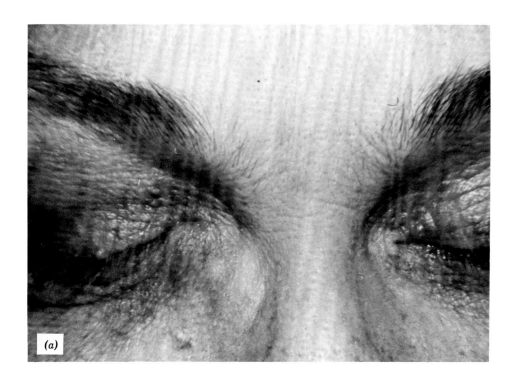

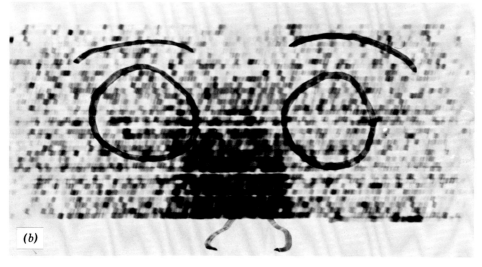

Fig. 24. (a) Lymphoma of lacrimal sac. (b) Scan demonstrates localized activity inferior-medial aspect right orbit.

SUMMARY

Tumors of the globe and orbit can be successfully localized and imaged by radionuclide techniques. These methods have been extensively investigated and are being utilized in many institutions.

Radioactive phosphorous is utilized for localization of intraocular melanomas employing Geiger-Mueller or semiconductor contact detectors. Noncontact detection techniques utilize ^{125}I- and ^{123}I-labeled chloroquine with specially designed pin-hole collimators. Other isotopes such as ^{197}Hg-chlormerodrin and ^{131}I-chloroquine have been utilized but are not as widely accepted.

Scanning and imaging techniques employing ^{197}Hg-chlormerodrin and ^{99m}Tc pertechnetate are now widely used in orbital tumor diagnosis.

Combined with x-ray examination of the skull and orbits these methods offer very satisfactory means for identifying and localizing suspected orbital malignancy.

REFERENCES

1. Duran-Reynals, F.: Studies on the Localization of Dyes and Foreign Proteins in Normal and Malignant Tissues. *Amer. J. Cancer* **35**:98 (1939).

2. Moore, G. E.: Fluorescein as an Agent in the Differentiation of Normal and Malignant Tissue. *Science* **106**:130 (1947).

3. Selverstone, B., Sweet, W. H., and Robinson, C. F.: Clinical Use of Radioactive Phosphorous in the Surgery of Brain Tumors. *Ann. Surg.* **130**:643 (1949).

4. Moore, G. E.: Use of Radioactive Diiodofluorescein in the Diagnosis and Localization of Brain Tumors, *Science* **107**:569 (1948).

5. Moore, G. E., Caudill, C. M., Marvin, J. F., Aust, J. B., Chou, S. N., and Smith, G. A.: Clinical and Experimental Studies of Intracranial Tumors with Fluorescein Dyes with an Additional Note Concerning the Possible Use of ^{42}K and Iodine-131 Tagged Human Albumin. *Amer. J. Roentgenol. Radium Therapy Nucl. Med.* **66**:1 (1951).

6. Blau, M. and Bender, M. A.: Radiomercury (^{203}Hg) Labeled Neohydrin: A New Agent for Brain Tumor Localization. *J. Nucl. Med. (Convention Issue)* **35** (1959).

7. Harper, P. V., Veck, R., Charleston, D., and Lathrope, K. A.: Optimization of the Scanning Method Using ^{99m}Tc. *Nucleonics* **22**(1):50 (1964).

8. Burrows, E. H.: The Clinical Utility of Brain Scanning in Nuclear Medicine. In *Progress in Nuclear Medicine,* Vol. 1, Karger, Basel and University Park Press, Baltimore, 1972, pp. 287–335.

9. Jones, A. E., Koslow, M., Johnston, G. S., and Ommaya, A. K.: Gallium-67 Citrate Scintigraphy of Brain Tumors. *Radiology* **105**:693–697 (December 1972).

10. Mamo, L., Nouel, J-P., Robert, J., Chai, N., and Houdart, R.: Use of Radioactive Bleomycin to Detect Malignant Intracranial Tumors. *J. Neurosurg.* **39**:735–741 (December 1973).

11. Fagan, J. A., and Cowan, R. J.: The Effect of Potassium Perchlorate on Uptake of Pertechnetate-Tc^{99m} in Choroid Plexus Papillomas: A Report of Two Cases. *J. Nucl. Med.* **12**:312–314 (June 1971).

12. Buttfield, I. H., Wrench, J. C., Adiseshan, N., and Arnold, J.: Intravenous Perchlorate in Brain Scanning: Effects on Choroid Plexus and Lesion Visibility. *J. Nucl. Med.* **14**:543–545 (July 1973).

13. Zimmerman, H. M.: The Ten Most Common Types of Brain Tumors. *Seminars Roentol.,* **6**:48 (January 1971).

14. Cushing, H., and Eisenhardt, L.: *Meningiomas.* Charles C. Thomas, Springfield, Illinois, 1938.

15. Overton, M. C., Snodgrass, S. R., and Haynie, F. P.: Brain Scans in Neoplastic Intracranial Lesions: Scanning with Chlormerodrin ^{203}Hg and Chlormerodrin ^{197}Hg. *J. Amer. Med. Assoc.* **192**:747 (1965).

16. Goodrich, J. K., and Tutor, F. T.: The Isotope Encephlogram in Brain Tumor Diagnosis. *J. Nucl. Med.* **6**:541 (1965).

17. Quinn, J. L., III: Cumulative Results of Five Years of Brain Scanning with Technetium [99]M. In Blahd, W. H., Ed, *Nuclear Medicine*. McGraw-Hill, New York, 1971, p. 255.

18. Kety, S. S., and Schmidt, C. F.: The Nitrous Oxide Method for Determination of Cerebral Blood Flow in Man: Theory, Procedure, and Normal Values. *J. Clin. Invest.* **27**:476 (1948).

19. Lassen, N. A.: Intra-Arterial Methods for Measurement of Regional Cerebral Blood Flow in Man. In Gilson, A. J. and Smoak, W. B., Eds., *Central Nervous System Investigation with Radionuclides*. Charles C. Thomas, Springfield, Illinois, 1971.

20. Strauss, H. W., James, A. E., Hurley, P. J., DeLand, F. H., Moses, D. C., and Wagner, H. N.: Nuclear Cerebral Angiography: Usefulness in the Differential Diagnosis of Cerebrovascular Disease and Tumor. *Arch. Intern. Med.* **131**:211–216 (1973).

21. Rosenthall, L.: Intravenous Dynamic Nucleography of the Brain. In Croll, M. N. and Brady, L. W., Eds., *Recent Advances in Nuclear Medicine*. Appleton-Century-Crofts, New York, 1966.

22. Rosenthall, L.: Intravenous and Intracarotid Radionuclide Cerebral Angiography. *Seminars Nucl. Med.* **1**:70–84, (January 1971).

23. Solomon, H. C., Thompson, L. J., and Pfeiffer, H. M.: Circulation of Phenolsulfonephthalein in the Cerebro-Spinal System. *J. Amer. Med. Assoc.* **79**:1014 (1922).

24. Riselbach, R. E., DiChiro, G., Freireich, E. J., and Rall, D. P.: Subarachnoid Distribution of Drugs After Lumbar Injections. *New Engl. J. Med.* **267**:1273 (1962).

25. DiChiro, G., Reames, P. M., and Matthews, W. B., Jr.: RISA-ventriculography and RISA-cisternography, *Neurology* **14**:185 (1964).

26. Harbert, J. C.: Radionuclide Cisternography. *Seminars Nucl. Med.* **1**:92 (January 1971).

27. Milhorat, Thomas H.: *Hydrocephalus and the Cerebrospinal Fluid*. Williams and Wilkins Company, Baltimore, 1972.

28. DeLand, F. H.: The Biological Behavior of [169]Yb-DTPA after Intrafecal Administration. *J. Nucl. Med.* **14**:93–98 (February 1973).

29. Oldham, R. K., and Staab, E. V.: Aseptic Meningitis Following the Intrafecal Injection of Radioiodinated Serum Albumin. *Radiology* **97**:317–321 (November 1970).

30. Alderson, P. O. and Siegel, D. A.: Adverse Reactions Following ^{111}In-DTPA Cisternography. *J. Nucl. Med.* **14**:609–611 (August 1973).

31. Larson, S. M., Schall, G. L., and DiChiro, G.: Influence of Previous Lumbar Puncture and Pneumoencephalography on Incidence of Unsuccessful Radioisotope Cisternography. *J. Nucl. Med.* **12**:555–557 (August 1971).

32. Larson, S. M., Schall, G. L., and DiCharo, G.: The Unsuccessful Injection in Cisternography; Incidence, Cause and Appearance. In Harbert, John C. Ed., *Cisternography and Hydrocephalus A Symposium*, Charles C Thomas, Springfield, Illinois, 1972, pp. 153–160.

33. Mamo, L., Cophignon, J., Rey, A., and Houdart, R.: Interet de la Cisternographic Isotopique Daus Le Diagnostic Des Tumeurs De L'Angle Ponto-Cere Belleux. *Presse Med.* **79**:627–630 (March 20, 1971).

34. Ommaya, A. K., DiChiro, G., Maitland, B., and Pennybacker, J.B.: Non-Traumatic Cerebrospinal Fluid Rhinorrhea. *J. Neurol. Neurosurg Psychiat.* **31**:214–225, (1968).

35. Bauer, F., and Yuhl, E.: Myelography by Means of [131]I: The Myeloscintigram. *Neurology* **3**:341–346 (1953).

36. Voutilainen, A., Paasio, J., and Pesonen, K.: Experiences with Myeloscintography. *Acta Neurol. Scand.* **45**:583–593 (1969).

37. DiChiro, G., Ashburn, W., and Briner, W.: Technetium [99m] Serum Albumin for Cisternography. *Arch. Neurol.* **19**:00 (August 1968).

38. Perryman, C., Noble, P., and Bragdon, F.: Myeloscintography: A Useful Procedure for Localization of Spinal Block Lesions. *Amer. J. Roentgenology*, **80**:104–111 (1958).

39. Blahd, W.: *Nuclear Medicine* 2nd ed., 1971, pp. 277–294. McGraw-Hill Book Co., N.Y.

40. Shields, J. A., and Zimmerman, L. E.: Lesions Simulating Malignant Melanoma of the Posterior Uvea. *Arch. Ophthalmol.*, **89**:6, 466–471 (1973).

41. Shields, J. A., McDonald, P. R.: Improvement in The Diagnosis of Posterior Uveal Melanomas. *Arch. Ophthalmol.* **91**:259–264 (1974).

42. Thomas, C. F., Krohmer, J. S., Storaasli, J. P.: Detection of Intraocular Tumors with Radioactive Phosphorous. *A.M.A. Arch. Ophthamol.* **47**:276–286 (1952).

43. Thomas, C. I., Krohmer, J. S., and Storaasli, J. P.: Geiger Counter Probe for Diagnosis and Localization of Posterior Intraocular Tumors. *A.M.A. Arch. Ophthalmol.* **52**:413–414 (1954).

44. Hagler, W. S., Jarrett, W. H., Humphrey, W. C.: Radioactive Phosphorous Uptake Test in Diagnosis of Uveal Melanoma. *Arch. Ophthalmol.* **83**:548–557 (1970).

45. Carmichael, P. L., Federman, J., Shields, J., and Holst, G.: Further Considerations of ^{32}P Studies in Ocular Melanomas. Presented at Association for Research in Vision and Ophthalmology, May 1973.

46. Carmichael, P. L., and Leopold, I. H.: The Radioactive Phosphorous Test in Ophthalmology. *Amer. J. Ophthalmol.* **49**:484–488 (1960).

47. Goldberg, B., Taboritz, O., Kara, G. B., Zavell, A. and Espiritu, R.: Use of ^{32}P in Diagnosis of Intraocular Tumors. *Amer. Med. Assoc. Arch. Ophthalmol.* **65**:196–211 (1961).

48. Thomas, C. I., Bovington, M. S., and Krohmer, J. S.: I. Comparison of Radioactivity in Neoplastic and Normal Ocular Tissue. *Cancer Res.* **16**:796–803 (1956).

49. Packer, S., Lange, R.: Radioactive Phosphorous for the Detection of Ocular Melanomas: A Critical Evaluation. *Arch. Ophthalmol.* **90**:17–20 (1973).

50. LaRose, J. H.: Semiconductor Detectors for Eye Tumor Diagnosis In Hoffer, P. B., Beck, R. N., and Gottschalk, A., Eds., *The Role of Semiconductor Detectors in the Future of Nuclear Medicine.* Society of Nuclear Medicine Inc., N.Y. p. 190–205, 1971.

51. Boyd, C. M., Beierwaltes, W. H., Lieberman, L. M. et al: ^{125}I Labeled Chloroquine Analog in the Diagnosis of Ocular Melanomas. *J. Nucl. Med.* **11**:303 (1970).

52. Packer, S., Wolf, A. P., Redoanly, C., Atkins, H. L., and Lambrecht, R. M.: A New Radiopharmaceutical for the Detection of Melanoma. Presented at the Association for Research in Vision and Ophthalmology, Sarasota, Florida, May 1973.

53. Verin, Ph., Blouquet, P., Safi, N., and Moretti, J. L.: Douvelles Applications des Isotopes dans le Diagnostic Ophthalmologique. *Bull. Soc. Ophthalmol., France* **70**:640–648 (1970).

54. Leopold, I. H., Keates, E. U., and Charkes, I. D.: Role of Isotopes in Diagnosis of Intraocular Neoplasm. *Trans. Amer. Ophthalmol. Soc.* **62**:89–99 (1964).

55. Brady, L. W., Croll, M. N., Carmichael, P. L., and Wallner, R. J.: Imaging Intraocular Tumors Utilizing Gallium-67 Citrate. Excerpta Medica XIII International Congress of Radiology 301, No. 978, Madrid, Spain, October 15–20, 1973.

56. Heuer, H. E., Ehlers, N., and Hansen, H. H.: La Scintigraphic des Tumerus Intraoculaires A L'Aide Du Ga-67. *Ann. Oculist (Paris)* **10**:1109–1113 (1972).

57. Greaves, D. P., and Cappin, J. M.: Mercury-197 Chlomerodrin in the Diagnosis of Intraocular Tumours. *Brit. J. Ophthalmol.* **56**:805–811 (1972).

58. Fillipone, C., Lenti, R., DeJulies, G., Morbiducci, G., and Muzzi, M.: Passibilita d'Impiego Della Scintigrafia Cerebrale per la Diagnosi di Affezioni Tumorali Oculari e Neuro-Oftalmiche Mediante Neo-Hydrin Marcato Cen ^{203}Hg. *Minerva Oftalmol.* **10**:234–261 (1968).

59. Hopping, W.: Augentumor-Diagnostik mit Gamma-Strahlern. *Bibliotheca Ophthalmol.* **75**:61–67 (1968).

60. Trokel, S. L., and Schlesinger, E. B., Beaton, H.: Diagnosis of Orbital Tumors by Gamma Ray Orbitography. *Amer. J. Ophthalmol.* **74**:675–679, (1972).

61. Flanagan, J.: Localization of Intraorbital Tumors with ^{99m}Technetium. Paper presented at Second International Symposium on Orbital Disorders. May 29–30, 1973.

62. Croll, M. N., Carmichael, P. L., Wallner, R. J., and Brady, L. W.: Localization of Orbital Tumors by Rectilinear Scanning with ^{99m}Tc and ^{197}Hg. Excerpta Medica XIII International Congress of Radiology 301, No. 978, Madrid, Spain, October 15–20, 1973.

63. Grove, A. S. Jr., Kotner, L. M. Jr.: Radionuclide Arteriography in Ophthalmology. *Arch. Ophthalmol.* **89**:13–17 (1973).

Discussion

Dr. Seydel. I would like to open the discussion by asking how new equipment such as the EMI x-ray transverse axial scanning tomograph fits in with the isotope techniques which have been mentioned.

Dr. David Kuhl. I think in view of the expense of the EMI system that our methods of studying brain tumors in most of the country will be much the same for some time. In the future we, of course, would like more information about how the EMI machine performs in sensitivity and specificity for the detection of tumors, but from the information that we have right now it appears that it is an extremely useful instrument for looking at the ventricles without the introduction of air, and for detecting some tumors that might not be easily detectable with brain scanning, for instance the craniopharyngiomas, lesions around the pituitary, and for looking at intracerebral hematomas and hemorrhage in the brain especially if they are of longer duration. Now from my own personal interest in this field, I would predict that a very powerful study method of the brain for the future will be in the cross sectional format where one looks at cross sectional density pictures of pertechnetate distribution reflecting blood–brain barrier alterations such as we have been doing with our transverse section scanning with pertechnetate, cross-section quantitative pictures of regional cerebral blood volume, regional cerebral blood flow and, if we are clever enough, regional cerebral metabolism. All of these pictures are done with an intravenous injection of material or no injection of material at all rather than with air contrast studies. I think the impact of these studies will not be to alter the use of the brain scan as a survey as it's done today, but to add considerably more information about patients who we know are abnormal to begin with. As far as I know there is no commercially available emission transverse section scanner. The EMI scanner is the only commercially available transmission scanner, but I do know that there is a lot of ferment in different companies around the world and I would expect that both kinds of machines will be commercially available from other companies.

Discussant. I just wondered if Dr. Kuhl would like to comment on new scanning agents like indium-labeled bleomycin.

Dr. Kuhl. In the brain or in other parts of the body?

Discussant. In the brain.

Dr. Kuhl. I think that labeled bleomycin and gallium are useful in selected patients, especially patients with metastatic disease. I think however that unfortunately the percentage of those who are positive is probably still down around 50% so that if your patient is positive with one of these agents he is very positive and this can be extremely useful information. However, the search for more effective agents of this type must continue.

Dr. Seymour Levin. Are you able to visualize chromophobe adenomas on scans or are these just sellar vascular lesions that you spoke about?

Dr. Kuhl. We were disappointed with the results of our section scanning when applying it to sellar lesions. Chromophobe adenomas were found in the sections if they had extended above the sella and extended into the third ventricle. In normal patients,

47

difficulty was encountered with blood in the cavernous sinus. The problem with conventional radionuclide scanning of pituitary lesions is that they are frequently cystic and, therefore, do not take up the isotope. The lesion alters the radiograph before it alters the scan, and the lesions that we generally found were already known to us before scanning.

Discussant.   I was going to ask if you think any of these techniques will distinguish solid pituitary lesions from cystic ones? We had high hopes that the EMI scanner might be useful in this respect, but to date it has been rather disappointing in making such a distinction of solid versus cystic lesions of the pituitary. Do any of the other techniques allow that? I would say that we have had some experience in our unit with an EMI scanner and my current appraisal is that it does little to replace the conventional in-patient diagnostic procedures of angiography and encephalography, but in my mind it is quite superior to what we have been accustomed to in the past for out-patient application.

Dr. Kuhl.   I have no experience at all with EMI scanning and I do not know of any other modality which could distinguish a cystic pituitary lesion from a solid one. I would be surprised if EMI scanning would have a large impact on the conventional use of radioisotope scanning. Isotope scanning is generally a survey of the total cerebral mass, and the EMI x-ray scans still require one to be selective in the planes of the brain which one wishes to display. In an equivalent amount of time, expense of dollars and effort, one could probably survey the brain more efficiently with four ordinary brain scans used in the search for tumor than with a multiplane EMI scan survey. I say this with ignorance of the EMI scan method, but it is difficult to study the whole volume of the brain with this type of modality.

Discussant.   I have only seen the EMI scanner as an outsider, but the normal technique with which it is applied is to do a series of sections so that the whole brain is reasonably well covered. I haven't been conscious of that as a substantial limitation.

The Surgical Approach to the Treatment of Gliomas

John F. Mullan, M.D.,
John Harper Seeley Professor
and Chairman of Neurosurgery,
University of Chicago
Hospitals and Clinics,
Chicago, Illinois

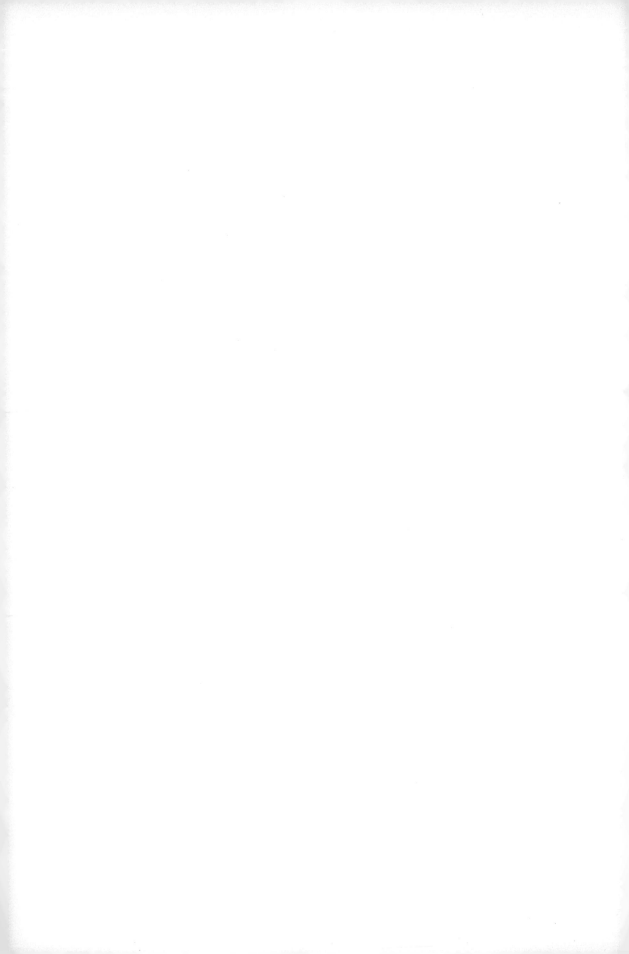

The Surgical Approach to the Treatment of Gliomas

John F. Mullan, M.D.,
John Harper Seeley Professor
and Chairman of Neurosurgery,
University of Chicago
Hospitals and Clinics,
Chicago, Illinois

Surgical treatment of brain tumors has now reached a point of technical evolution at which its goals and accomplishments can be fairly accurately assessed. The associated mortality that stood about 50% at the turn of the century has now virtually disappeared.[13] Morbidity incurred as surgeons strove toward a "cure" in every case has receded with the realization that the realistic goal of surgical management in many instances is that of palliation. It seems unlikely that technical developments in the surgical art will greatly increase the effectiveness of surgical treatment, but it is quite possible that new methods of diagnosis will discover smaller earlier tumors and will thereby considerably improve results.

Recent improvements in morbidity, mortality, and results have been largely due to earlier diagnosis, safer diagnosis, and especially to better control of intracranial pressure. Accurate hemostasis, better anesthesia, cortisone in cortisone-deficient states, regulation of fluids, and the availability of antibiotics have long been taken for granted.

Early diagnosis depends largely upon the greater numbers of trained neurologists, neurosurgeons, and neuroradiologists now in practice and in teaching. It also depends upon the early and widely available use of brain scanning, which yields positive information in more than 80% of tumor cases even when the location is in the posterior fossa.[12] The detection of technetium by the newer scintillation cameras compares favorably with the results of more conventional angiography. While it is true that angiography will detect some very slowly growing avascular or cystic tumors not seen by the camera, it is apparent that the camera will detect many small and deep lesions that are missed by angiography.

Thus today's patient rarely presents with an instantly life-threatening situation and there is time for a thorough medical evaluation that will uncover and treat cardiac, pulmonary, renal, and metabolic defects. Widespread acceptance that lumbar puncture is an unnecessary and potentially dangerous test has all but eliminated the once familiar brain stem herniation during investigation (if a brain tumor is suspected the problem should be totally evaluated whether the lumbar pressure is high or low). Control of intracranial pressure before pneumoencephalography or ventriculography, has eliminated the once customary practice of rushing into surgery upon completion of the test lest consequent herniation should develop. Angiography, whether performed by carotid puncture or by femoral catheter, carries a risk related almost entirely to the technique of needle or catheter insertion. Subintimal carotid injection in a patient who cannot tolerate carotid occlusion can be catastrophic. It is much more dangerous than the subsequent craniotomy. The problem is solved by ensuring that only the most skilled individual carries out the test in all high-risk patients. With this precaution the risk is virtually zero. It is true that contrast material may leak into areas with deficient blood–brain barrier offering a possible risk. In these situations the volume of injection should be kept to a minimum. Allergic reactions to iodine should be prevented by a knowledge of previous difficulty or of allergy to shellfish.

PREOPERATIVE CONTROL OF PRESSURE

General surgeons have long since recognized the hazards of operating upon the obstructed gut and will, if possible, carry out a decompression procedure before undertaking a definitive excision. The same principle should apply to neurosurgical obstructions. When raised intracranial pressure is diagnosed clinically, control of the local brain swelling around some tumors, especially metastatic tumors and

51

glioblastomas, should be initiated early by the use of dexamethasone (16 mg daily). When cerebrospinal fluid obstruction by a suspected posterior fossa tumor, aqueduct, or third ventricle lesion is diagnosed it should be relieved by a ventriculo-caval shunt before ventriculography is performed.[5] In some acute situations urea or mannitol will control pressure for a few hours or even a day or two while diagnostic and operative preparations are completed.

Operation upon a slack rather than a tense brain is technically simpler and therefore safer, requiring less retraction and affording easier hemostasis. In nonresectable supratentorial infiltrating tumors involving the central or speech areas, a simple biopsy may be taken without requiring either an internal or an external decompression. In posterior fossa tumors the improvements brought about through control of pressure (through preoperative shunting) are even more spectacular. For tumors such as medulloblastomas or solid hemangiomas a safe and simple biopsy may be accomplished without laboring in an impossible therapeutic situation merely to unblock the aqueduct. In posterior fossa tumors the once familiarly distressing postoperative period, presumably associated with the difficulties of a blood-laden CSF finding its absorption pathways, is no longer observed. Posterior fossa wound-bulging is not apparent. Convalescence is rapid. In the author's opinion this preoperative shunting has made posterior fossa surgery as simple and safe as supratentorial surgery.

PLANNING THE EXTENT OF SURGERY

Exploratory intracranial surgery no longer exists. The exact position, blood supply, and blood drainage must be known in advance, and not infrequently the angiogram, scan, site, and clinical presentation have given the surgeon accurate knowledge as to histological type. With this information he must plan the precise extent of his removal. He must decide before surgery if the patient can survive total extirpation and if the consequent neurological deficit is acceptable. If these considerations force him to consider subtotal resection he must then decide upon the extent of operation that will relieve symptoms and prolong life in the most meaningful manner. There is no point in performing a subtotal operation that will increase symptoms. In some instances he should decide to wait until presenting symptoms exceed or equal the anticipated deficit.

Since infiltrating white-matter tumors in most instances destroy the connections to the overlying gray, the carotid mantle is in fact functionless. Lobectomy rather than a removal confined to the tumor itself is therefore the preferable procedure in that it will provide greater decompression without additional deficit. In some cystic and slowly growing gliomas, white matter and overlying gray are displaced rather than infiltrated and these may be enucleated. In general, removal of infiltrated motor strip or speech areas does not provide meaningful palliation. If the bulk of these central tumors is a problem, it is best to confine removal to the adjoining lobe that is most densely infiltrated. Rarely, with speech cortex, a subtemporal decompression is still applicable. Infiltrating tumors of the anterior and posterior perforated areas, the hypothalamus, the brain stem, and medulla are not surgically removable without catastrophic disability or death. Rarely a cyst of these areas may be aspirated.

CORTICAL LOCALIZATION

At operation the surgeon has a fairly good idea of the motor strip and speech areas by simple inspection. This, however, is not good enough; a 1-cm error could be catastrophic. Motor area can be simply mapped by electrical stimulation in the lightly anesthetized patient (2–5 V, 2-mc duration, 60-cycle square waves). The sensory area can be mapped by evoked potentials using an averaging computer or by inference from the motor area. The speech areas can be outlined by operating under local anesthesia. Electrical stimulation of the cortex supresses speech. Accurate knowledge of these areas allows the surgeon to remove the maximum amount of tumor safely.

BIOPSY

It has been customary to advise biopsy for tumors that cannot be removed. This is a general principle in cancer surgery before beginning radiotherapy. Intracranial needle biopsy is not applicable to the brain stem, and its wisdom in many instances of glioblastoma is open to question. Serious hemorrhage can occur. In some of these the clinical, isotope, and angiographic diagnosis is so typical that no other diagnosis need be considered before instituting radiotherapy. In the majority where diagnosis is not so clear, it is better to make an open biopsy through a small bone flap with full antipressure precautions. Accurate localization and good control of pressure preoperatively by cortisone or shunting and intraoperatively by urea or mannitol make this a safer though more arduous procedure than blind needle biopsy.

SURGICAL RESULTS

The virtual disappearance of neurosurgical mortality and morbidity has been taken for granted by neurosurgeons, but few have commented upon this in the literature.[13] Current reports deal mainly with unusual tumors collected over many years or unusual types of common tumor. Consequently, the mortality figures quoted do not reflect the present state of the art but rather the average figures over 30 or 40 years of development. They may give an erroneous impression of the present state of this surgical treatment. However, these reviews do give a fairly good example of the long-term results to be expected in those patients who survived the earlier operative methods.

ASTROCYTE SERIES

The ability of a cerebral tumor to cause death or disability depends both upon its rate of growth and upon its exact location. Its future rate of growth can be estimated both by the histological appearance and by its clinical course. Thus, in planning treatment, evaluating results, and assessing the literature one must consider cell type, location, and clinical history of growth.

Histological categories of gliomas are somewhat arbitrary whether we follow Kernahan's four groups of malignancy or Elvidge's five cell groups—piloid astrocytoma, gemistocytic astrocytoma, astrocytoma diffusum, glioblastoma multiforme, and a miscellaneous group that fits in between astrocytoma diffusum and glioblastome. If we lump astrocytoma diffusum and gemistocytic astrocytoma together and regard them as group 2 we end up roughly with Kernahan's four groups. For a relatively modern careful long-term followup of a significant number of cases we might consider Elvidge's recent review.[2]

Piloid (group 1). Often cystic, occur frequently in the cerebellum but also in the cerebrum. In the midline cerebellum they occur at a younger age (about 12) in contrast to the average age of 31.5. Out of 34 patients, 7 deaths (3 cystic) occurred between 6 and 30 years later. One had x-ray treatment in addition to surgical removal. Fourteen (12 cystic) were still alive between 13 and 38 years later. One of these had radiation. Six had mitotic figures at the time of surgery. Thus long-term survival and even cure may be expected. Radiation as given was probably not of value. Mitotic figures did not contraindicate good prognosis.

Astrocytoma diffusum (group 2 approximately). The average age of survival of 19 patients was over 5 years and the longest survival was more than 18 years. Mitosis was unfavorable but did not preclude long-term survival. Five of the 8 long-term survivors had x-ray, as did 6 of the 17 shorter survivors.

Gemistocytic astrocytomas (group 2 approximately). Out of 26 cases the average survival was just less than 4 years and the longest just over 10 years. Five cases had x-ray therapy without obvious change in survival. Three who showed mitosis belonged to the longer survivals, though in general the presence of mitosis was less favorable.

Elvidge's miscellaneous group (group 3 approximately). For 112 patients, survival with surgery was 28 months, but with added radiation it was 43 months.

Glioblastomas (group 4). The average survival for 399 patients was 9.8 months, but with added radiation it was 17.4 months. Two patients survived 19 and 25 years. The latter, who died of a heart attack, did not have radiation.

Roth and Elvidge in a previous communication reported little difference in survival between those patients who had a total removal and those who had a subtotal removal.[15] Jelsma and Bucy on the other hand have strongly advocated radical removals.[8] They believe this policy resulted in a lowered operative mortality and gave some longer survivors. Of 162 patients, 10 lived more than 2 years. Over the period 1945–1967 their operative mortality dropped from 48 to 2.8%. The two factors of importance in reducing this were, in their opinion, more extensive removals and the use of dexamethasone.

BRAIN STEM GLIOMA

Elvidge's report of piloid astrocytes of the brain stem with a survival of 1.5 years represents the classical opinion as to longevity, but those series that include all varieties of glioma may be expected to have an even worse prognosis. Surgical exploration or treatment as a rule is not advised except in unusual situations to relieve cerebrospinal fluid obstruction. Lassiter has recently pointed out that cysts exist in some of these patients.[10] In a series of 25 who survived exploration, 6 lived 7.5 years or longer. Four (2 still living) had large cysts. All had x-ray treatment. It was believed that drainage of these cysts contributed to the relatively good survivals.

OPTIC CHIASM GLIOMAS

This is a very slowly growing tumor that resembles the piloid astrocytoma of the cerebellum. It is rarely ammenable to radical removal. Occasionally a cyst can be evacuated. If obstruction of a third ventricle occurs a Torkildsen shunt is required. Because of the slow growth of these tumors it has been difficult to evaluate radiation, but current evidence favors it. Taveras noted improvement in 4 of 17 patients.[21] McCarty in a series of 20 patients carried out excision in 7 and biopsy and radiation in 13.[11] Five of these 13 showed objective improvement, 2 remained static over 8 and 10 years followup. The remainder deteriorated. Two of these have since died. It would appear that this very slowly growing tumor may preserve vision for a very long time. Radiotherapy has an established place in treatment. It is not entirely certain that surgical excision of gliomas confined to a single optic nerve is useful since evidence is still lacking that these tumors spread or metastasize if left undisturbed. In most neurosurgeons' clinical practice the proportion of tumors that could be resected is probably much smaller than in McCarty's.

OLIGODENDRO GLIOMAS

These somewhat slowly growing tumors, situated mostly in the frontal lobes have, in the review by Weir and Elvidge of 63 cases, a rather favorable prognosis.[22] Forty one percent survived more than 5 years. Thirty were still alive at followup. Of those who died, the average survival was 4 years. Of those who have since died following a total resection, survival was 6.8 years. Weir and Elvidge used radiotherapy but did not evaluate it. Roberts and German, reviewing Cushing's 38 cases, reported a mortality of 10%.[14] The average duration of survival was 5.6 years and the longest was 36, this patient being still alive at the time of reporting. Those with a total removal had an average survival of 13 years. In 21 who had radiation, survival was 6.8 years. In those who did not it was 5.2 years. Thus both tend to favor total removal and, to a lesser extent, radiotherapy. Shenken,[16] who preferred radiotherapy at the time of tumor recurrence, showed that 4 patients treated at this stage developed remission of serious symptoms and 3 returned to fully useful lives.

EPENDYMOMA

Barone and Elvidge reviewed 47 intracranial and 27 intraspinal tumors.[1] They attempted surgical removal in 27 patients and believed it was complete in 16. Nine were alive between 2 and 21 years afterwards. Three of the remaining 7 died of other causes. The 12-year average survival of those patients in whom the tumor was completely removed was contrasted with an 8-year average survival of those in whom it was partially removed. Partial removal without x-ray gave a survival of 2.5 years, but with x-ray it was 9.5 years. Of those still alive after 18 years, 4 had incomplete removals without x-ray and 2 had incomplete removals with x-ray. The operative mortality was 31.9%. It would appear therefore that ependymomas benefit from total removal where applicable and from x-ray therapy when removal is subtotal.

Fokes and Earl in a review of 180 cases commented upon the difficulties in grading these tumors, but believe that infratentorial tumors, which are more common (69%), were less malignant than those above the tent.[4] Survivals (excluding postoperative deaths) averaged 32.9 months for infratentorial tumors and 41.3 months for the supratentorial group. With added radiotherapy the survivals were 53.2 and 16.1 months, respectively. Kricheff reviewed the literature and reporting on 65 cases stated that the prognosis was poorer in children than in adults, that radiotherapy was a useful agent, and that there was no justification for irradiating the entire axis.[9] His patients with infratentorial lesions survived 6 years and with supratentorial lesions they survived 2.8 years.

MEDULLOBLASTOMA

It is generally assumed that this is a tumor of childhood with a dismal prognosis. A few similar tumors in adults (regarded by some as leptomeningeal sarcomas) have only a slightly better outlook. Since in most instances surgical management is confined to obtaining a biopsy, this is an ideal situation for shunting. The surgeon does not then need to engage in extensive surgery and in the high attending mortality and morbidity merely to unblock the aqueduct but takes a simple surface biopsy. In the review of Smith et al the operative mortality was 20%.[18] They did, however, offer a more optimistic note on the results of radiotherapy. There was a 28% 5-year survival. The quality of survival in the earlier patients subjected to intensive local irradiation was poor, but improvement was seen in those given a more prolonged and much wider field of therapy. Hope-Stone, using a homogenous total nervous system radiation technique, reported upon a 75% 5-year survival and upon a 50% 10-year survival in a limited number of cases.[6] There were 10 in his 10-year series.

PINEALOMA

The mixed group of tumors in the pineal region include germinomas, teratomas, true pineal cell tumors, and gliomas. It has been generally accepted that operative mortality was prohibitive, that those with the more benign tumors did well with shunting (ventriculo cistern anastomosis), that the radiosensitive group (probably 70% of the total) did reasonably well with radiation and shunting, and that those who did not respond to radiation and shunting probably had tumors that were so malignant that not much could be done for them surgically. Recently Suzuki and Iwabuchi,[20] Stein,[19] and Jamieson[7] have reconsidered the possibility of excision, the last two authors having no mortality in a series of 6 cases each. DeGirolami and Schmidek reviewed 53 cases over a 42-year period and reported a biopsy–removal mortality of 33–60%.[3] They believe that only in very selected instances should surgery be preferred to the traditional shunt and radiation treatment. These cases are probably those with teratomas, pineocytomas, or cysts that showed progressive but slow growth after having had shunt and radiotherapy. Those patients with germinomas showed a 10-year average survival after surgery and radiation and the pathologically unverified group (having had no biopsy) had a 4-year survival.

HEMANGIOMA

This somewhat rare tumor is most common in the cerebellum. It may be cystic or solid and may or may not involve the brain stem. It may be associated with polycythemia. Shige-Hisa reported that 19 patients over a 30-year period had an operative mortality of 50% in the solid tumors and 15% in the cystic. These figures reflect problems not now encountered.[17] Preoperative shunting would have avoided the pneumoencephalographic, the ventriculographic, and the extreme-brain-swelling deaths. Preoperative angiography and scanning would have localized those within the brain stem that should not have been resected. The response of some of these to simple decompression was good. Recent information on radiotherapy is sparse.

COLLOID CYST OF THE THIRD VENTRICLE

This is the simplest of all brain tumors to remove and the operation should be accomplished without mortality or morbidity by the transventricular approach.

PAPILLOMA OF THE CHOROIDAL PLEXUS

Wilkins report of 19 cases with a mortality of 25% would also suggest that much of this difficulty could now be avoided by preoperative shunting since the tumors are essentially benign.[23]

DISCUSSION

This survey of the recent neurosurgical literature is not inclusive. It is merely a selection of a few of the larger series. The mortality of those extending over earlier years reflects the rather catastrophic figures of those years.[3, 17] However, the more recent reports clearly show that even with admittedly difficult tumors a low figure may be obtained such as the zero by Jamieson[7] and Stein[19] for pinealomas and the 2.3% by Jelsma and Bucy for glioblastomas. In 1962 the author reported 3 postoperative deaths in a consecutive series of 100 brain tumors.[13] Two followed biopsy of glioblastomas. Greater attention to the peculiar problems of hemostasis associated with this procedure has eliminated the intratumor hematoma that was responsible for slow deterioration of both these patients. The third of the series died of acute hepatitis associated with homologous serum jaundice. A more meticulous hemostatic technique since that time has all but eliminated the need for blood transfusion with its consequent risk of induced viral infection. The easy availability of blood had probably led to overtransfusion in the past. It is not imperative that each patient finish surgery with the same hematocrit he had at the beginning. In fact it should be remembered that pulmonary embolism is rare if the hematocrit is below 30. In the 11 years subsequent to that report the author has not had any mortality in the surgical management of gliomas. It is his opinion that meticulous preoperative, operative, and postoperative control of intracranial pressure by dexamethasone, urea, mannitol, and shunting is the single most important factor in maintaining a consistently low mortality and complication rate.

A study of the long-term followup is complicated by the lack of a uniform method of reporting. Average survival times, 5-year survival rates, and longest survival times have all been used. The fact that a substantial number of patients are still living in many of the series adds further to the incompleteness of the picture. Failure to set up prospective studies of radiotherapy diminish the usefulness of the evaluation of this therapeutic method. Despite these many problems a fairly good picture of the prognosis following surgery does emerge.

The most benign astrocytoma has a reasonably good chance of surviving a decade and may survive four decades or more. Most recurrences occur early, but a few occur later and a few may undergo a more malignant change. Long-term survival is possible even when removal is incomplete. There is no information that radiotherapy has a role.

The next group of astrocytomas (group 2) has an average survival of 4–5 years and a long-term survival of 10–18 years. The astrocytoma diffusion is more favorable than the gemistocytic tumor. The role of radiotherapy is uncertain. In group 3 astrocytomas a surgical survival greater than 2 years was extended beyond 3 years by added radiation, while with glioblastomas a survival of 0.75 year was extended to 1.5 years by radiation. There was conflicting opinion as to the value of extensive surgical removal in terms of long survival, though it would appear to occupy a prominant position in lowering immediate mortality.

In the management of brain stem gliomas a new idea has appeared[10]—surgical exploration with evacuation of cysts. It remains to be developed. Attention has also been drawn to the possibility of some long-term survivals of 7 years or more. Radiation (and biopsy) would appear to be effective in one-half of the treated patients with optic nerve glioma who either improved or remained static, with at least one remaining static over 10 years. A few selected patients with gliomas confined to one optic nerve may have total excision.

The outlook for oligodendrogliomas is that of a 5.5-year average survival, somewhat increased by radiation. In fact, in a few instances when radiation only was used in the face of recurrence it was quite clearly effective. The longest reported survival was 36 years. Ependymomas offer about a 3-year average survival with surgery and one of 4–9 years with added radiation. Total removal was preferable to partial. There was conflicting opinion as to the importance of the location relative to the tentorium.

The outlook for those with medulloblastoma has been considerably brightened by the reports[17, 18] that radiotherapy can achieve a 5-year survival of greater than 50%. It would appear that preoperative shunting, minimal biopsy, and radiotherapy offer the best available help. A new look has been taken at the possibility of direct surgical removal of selected pineal tumors by master surgeons. The key words here are "selected" and "master." Any attempt to make this a routine procedure would simply reinstate the dismal experience recounted by DeGirolami and Schmidek.[3] Ventriculo cisternostomy and radiation remain the initial and standard treatment. Hemangioma of the cerebellum, while not a glioma, has been discussed as an example of a tumor of the posterior fossa that should, in many instances, be shunted before being tackled surgically.

SUMMARY

A review of selected recent reports on the surgical treatment of gliomas notes that an operative mortality approaching zero has been reported in some of the more difficult tumors. It is suggested that meticulous control of intracranial pressure is a most important factor. The value of preoperative shunting in cases of obstruction of the cerebrospinal fluid is discussed. Some more recent ideas in management include surgical removal of pineal tumors and aspiration of brain stem glioma cysts. Long-term surveys of treated cases now give a fairly good idea of the results to be expected for each histological type.

REFERENCES

1. Barone, B. M., and Elvidge, A. R.: Ependymomas. A Clinical Survey. *J. Neurosurg.* **33:**428–438 (1970).

2. Elvidge, A. R.: Long-Term Survival in the Astrocytoma Series. *J. Neurosurg.* **28:**399–404 (1968).

3. DeGerolami, U., and Schmidek, H.: Clinicopathological Study of 53 Tumors of the Pineal Region. *J. Neurosurg.* **39:**455–462 (1973).

4. Fokes, E. C., and Earle, K. M.: Ependymomas: Clinical and Pathological Aspects. *J. Neurosurg.* **30:**585–594 (1969).

5. Hekmatpanah, J., and Mullan, S.: Ventriculo-Caval Shunt in the Management of Posterior Fossa Tumors. *J. Neurosurg.* **26:**609–613 (1967).

6. Hope-Stone, H. F.: Results of Treatment of Medulloblastomas. *J. Neurosurg.* **32:**83–88 (1970).

7. Jamieson, K. G.: Excision of Pineal Tumors. *J. Neurosurg.* **35:**550–553 (1971).

8. Jelsma, R., and Bucy, P. C.: The Treatment of Glioblastoma Multiforme of the Brain. *J. Neurosurg.* **27:**388–400 (1967).

9. Kricheff, I. I., Becker, M., Schneck, S. A., and Taveras, J. M.: Intracranial Ependymomas: Factors Influencing Prognosis. *J. Neurosurg.* **21:**7–14 (1964).

10. Lassiter, K. R. L., Alexander, E., Davis, C., and Kelly, D. L.: Surgical Treatment of Brain Stem Gliomas. *J. Neurosurg.* **34:**719–725 (1971).

11. MacCarty, C. S., Boyd, A. S., and Childs, D. S.: Tumors of the Optic Nerve and Optic Chiasm. *J. Neurosurg.* **33:**439–444 (1970).

12. Moody, R. A., Olsen, J. O., Gottschalk, A., and Hoffer, P. B.: Brain Scans of the Posterior Fossa. *J. Neurosurg.* **36:**148–152 (1972).

13. Mullan, S.: Current Mortality of the Surgical Treatment of Brain Tumors. *J. Amer. Med. Assoc.,* **182:**601–608 (1962).

14. Roberts, M., and German, W. J.: A Long Term Study of Patients with Oligodendrogliomas. *J. Neurosurg.* **24:**697–700 (1966).

15. Roth, J. G., and Elvidge, A. R.: Glioblastoma Multiforme: A Clinical Survey. *J. Neurosurg.* **17:**736–750 (1960).

16. Shenkin, H. A.: The Effect of Roentgen-Ray Therapy on Oligodendrogliomas of the Brain. *J. Neurosurg.* **22:**57–59 (1965).

17. Shige-Hisa, O.: Solid Cerebellar Hemangioblastoma. *J. Neurosurg.* **39:**514–518 (1973).

18. Smith, R. A., Lampe, I., and Kahn, E. A.: The Prognosis of Medulloblastoma in Children. *J. Neurosurg.* **18:**91–97 (1961).

19. Stein, B. M.: The Infratentorial Supracerebellar Approach to Pineal Lesions. *J. Neurosurg.,* **35:**197–202 (1971).

20. Suzuki, J., and Iwabuchi, T.: Surgical Removal of Pineal Tumors (Pinealomas and Teratomas) Experience in a Series of 19 Cases. *J. Neurosurg.* **23:**565–571 (1965).

21. Taveras, J. M., Mount, L. A., and Wood, E. H.: The Value of Radiation Therapy in the Management of Gliomas of the Optic Nerves and Chiasm. *Radiology* **66:**518–528 (1956).

22. Weir, B., and Elvidge, A.: Oligodendrogliomas: An Analysis of 63 Cases. *J. Neurosurg.* **29:**500–505 (1968).

23. Wilkins, H. and Rutledge, B. J.: Papillomas of the choroid plexus. *J. Neurosurg.* **18:**14–18 (1961).

Treatment of Glioblastoma Multiforme

Melvin L. Griem, M.D.,

Professor and Chairman,
Division of Radiation Therapy,
Chicago Tumor Institute of the
University of Chicago,
Chicago Illinois

Wai-Kwan Yung, B.Sc.,

American Cancer Society
Student Fellow,
Illinois Division,
Chicago, Illinois

J. E. Marks, M.D.,

American Cancer Society
Junior Faculty Fellow,
Division of Radiation Therapy,
Chicago Tumor Institute of the
University of Chicago,
Chicago, Illinois

William Steward, M.D.,

Professor of Radiology,
University of Chicago,
Director, Chicago Tumor
Institute of the University
of Chicago,
Chicago, Illinois

John F. Mullan, M.D.,

John Harper Seely
Professor and Chairman
of Neurosurgery,
University of Chicago
Hospitals and Clinics,
Chicago, Illinois

S uit has estimated that in patients with brain tumors, the principal reason for failure to cure by any means is the failure of local tumor control of this primary tumor.[11] Glioblastoma multiforme accounts for over 25% of all intracranial tumors. Much work has been done in the search for a treatment method that will lead to increased survival in these patients. Radical surgery results in morbidity and disability. Average survival is found to be about 30 weeks following surgery. Current treatment of choice is extensive surgical resection of the tumor mass in combination with postoperative megavoltage irradiation.[7, 8] Presently chemotherapeutic agents are being used in various combinations with surgery and radiation[13, 1] but marked improvement in survival has not been shown. Recent studies of the use of 1-3-bis(2-chloroethyl)-1-nitrosourea (BCNU) and radiation indicated a significant improvement in survival (Table 1).[12] At this symposium Chang presented his data showing the improvement in survival when patients are treated with radiation and high-pressure oxygen.[2] Because of the recent interest in the treatment of glioblastoma multiforme, we decided to evaluate the therapeutic results of various treatment techniques at The University of Chicago.

MATERIALS AND METHODS

All patients with the diagnosis of glioblastoma multiforme were evaluated for the period 1953–1971. The following materials were carefully reviewed: patient records, all radiologic studies, special arteriograms and pneumoencephalograms, the pathology report, and the histologic slides. All available histologic slides were examined by two observers, and efforts were made to confirm whether or not the tumors were glioblastoma multiforme. One hundred and fifteen patients were considered eligible for the study. Initially, three investigators, Yung, Marks, and Steward, evaluated the above material and recorded the data. The age, sex, location of the tumor, presenting signs and symptoms, x-ray studies, sintographic findings, the pathologic report, and histologic slides were reviewed and recorded. These results were correlated with the survival and change in status of the patient before and after treatment was recorded. These patients were divided into 6 groups according to treatment received: (1) no treatment after diagnosis; (2) radiation only, 5000–6000 rads the whole brain, daily treatment 5 days per week, 200 rads per fraction; (3) surgery only; (4) surgical resection plus postoperative irradiation, 5000–6000 rads whole brain radiation, 200 rads per fraction, daily treatment 5 days per week; (5) surgical resection, irradiation, and colchicine;[3] (6) surgical resection, irradiation, and induction of hyperthyroid state by administration of L-triiodothyronine.

During the interval between 1960 and 1963, a subpopulation of 18 patients who were eligible because of their good physical condition for the induction of a hyperthyroid state were treated with whole brain radiation while being hyperthyroid. These patients were consecutive referrals insofar as they were considered suitable candidates for this metabolic change. From 1963 onward, the treatment technique returned to that of radiation therapy of the whole brain as outlined under 4 above.

The hyperthyroid state was induced while the patients were hospitalized on a metabolic ward under the careful observation of a team of endocrinologists.* The

* The authors wish to express their gratitude and thanks particularly to the support of Dr. Richard Landau, Chairman of Endocrinology, Dr. Ann Lawrence, and Dr. Edward Ehrlich for their patience and their careful management of these 18 patients.

TABLE 1   GLIOBLASTOMA MULTIFORME
TREATED WITH BCNU

	No. of Patients	Median Survival
		(weeks)
Control	45	17
BCNU alone	45	20
Irradiation alone	45	28
Irradiation and BCNU	45	41

[a] All patients received conventional neurosurgery.

management consisted of administration of very large doses of L-triiodothyronine. Twenty-five microgram tablets were used and a dose of 500–1000 μg was administrated daily. The induction started with 300 μg, and daily doses were increased by 50–100 μg until the desired hyperthyroid state was achieved. At a basal metabolic rate of between +20 and +30, radiation therapy was started with the usual fractionated technique. Each of the 18 patients received a total tissue dose of 4000–4200 rads on the advice of Dr. J. W. J. Carpender, who suggested that true sensitization of the radiation effect by the hyperthyroid state would be demonstrated by the effectiveness of a lower total dose. After the completion of therapy, the triiodothronine was immediately stopped, and the patients were discharged from the hospital usually 3–5 days after the cessation of radiation therapy and hormone administration.

RESULTS

After careful review of all patient records, radiologic films, and histologic slices, 115 patients were included in this study. The three investigators reviewing the material initially classified the patients without knowledge of the method of treatment.

Among the 115 patients, 55 had postmortem examinations; in 8 cases, the diagnosis was based upon changes shown in the arteriograms without histologic studies. In some patients the lesion was located in a critical section of the brain where biopsy would have resulted in serious neurological disturbance. Attempts were made to review all histologic slides in the 107 cases that had biopsies, autopsies, or both; 81 cases were available and reviewed. The criteria employed in Kernohan's classification of astrocytoma[9] were used as a reference in the review of the slides. The tumors were carefully evaluated according to the degree of cellularity, pleomorphism, and anaplasia present, the prominence of vascular changes, the extent of any regressive changes such as hemorrhage and necrosis, the presence of giant cells, and the number of mitotic figures seen per high-powered field. On the basis of these factors, a histologic grade was then assigned. In 7 cases there was evidence of leptomeningeal spread and in 1 patient seeding in the subarachnoid space of the spinal cord was evident. Table 2 shows the grading of the tumors in each treatment group. Since only astrocytoma grades III and IV are considered to be glioblastoma multiforme,[9] all tumors of grades lower than III were excluded. Among the 81 tumors reviewed, 65 were grade IV, 11 were grade III, and in 5 cases the tumors showed a transition from grade III to grade IV. Based on ar-

TABLE 2. HISTOPATHOLOGY OF THE BIOPSY AND AUTOPSY SPECIMENS STUDIED

Type of Treatment[a]	−III	IV	Astrocytoma Grade Borderline (III–IV)	Total Number of Cases Studied
None	1	9	1	
	1	1	0	13
Radiation only	0	5	0	
	0	1	0	6
Surgery only	3	7	1	
	1	8	0	20
Radiation and surgery	2	4	1	
	0	13	1	21
Radiation, surgery, and colchicine	0	4	0	
	0	4	0	8
Radiation, surgery, and T_3	2	6	1	
	1	3	0	13
Total	11	65	5	81

[a] The upper row of numbers for each type of treatment refers to autopsy specimens. The lower row of numbers refers to surgical biopsy specimens.

teriographic and sintographic findings plus the history, the remaining patients were categorized as glioblastoma.

Figure 1 shows the mean survival of all patients treated with surgery and radiation and the 18 patients who, in addition, received triiodothyronine. This figure suggested further evaluation of the various treatment techniques used. Table 3 shows the survival

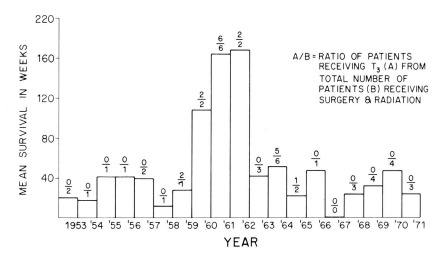

Fig. 1.   Mean survival of all patients treated with surgery and radiation, including those treated with T_3.

TABLE 3.   MEAN SURVIVAL OF PATIENTS IN EACH TREATMENT GROUP

Type of Treatment	Number of Cases	Shortest Survival (weeks)	Longest Survival (weeks)	Mean Survival (weeks)
None	23	1	14	5.0 ± 1.8
Radiation only	10	8	92	27.8 ± 18
Surgery only	24	1	36	5.6 ± 3.4
Radiation and surgery	32	4	74	31.7 ± 6.5
Radiation, surgery, and colchicine	8	2	68	35.8 ± 16
Radiation, surgery, and T_3[a]	18	26	360	106.3 ± 52
			(140)[b]	(60.3 ± 17)

[a] Triiodothyronine.
[b] Excluding 3 long survivors: 304, 352, and 360 weeks.

of the patients with each treatment method. As indicated, the group receiving surgery, radiation, and triiodothyronine had an unusually long survival, namely, 106 weeks mean survival as compared with the group receiving surgery and radiation, which has a survival of 31.6 weeks. Among the 18 patients receiving triiodothyronine, 3 survived for long periods of time—304 weeks, 352 weeks, and 360 weeks. If these 3 patients are excluded, the mean survival of this group becomes 60.3 weeks, which is still significantly better ($p = .005$) than that of the group receiving surgery and radiation.

The location and extent of involvement of each tumor were carefully recorded and tabulated. The most common location site was the frontal lobe from which these tumors often extended into the parietal and temporal lobes. Many tumors involved all four lobes of the cerebral hemisphere, which confirms the highly malignant and infiltrative nature of these neoplasms. Other tumors frequently involved the corpus callosum and extended into the opposite hemisphere. There was no significant difference in the location and extent of involvement of the tumors in each treatment group.

Of the 115 patients, 60% were male and 40% were female. The incidence of glioblastoma in this series was in the age group 50–59. The age distribution does show that the group receiving triiodothyronine was relatively younger than the other group.

With the discovery of the increased survival of the patients with triiodothyronine and radiation treatment, special attention was paid to the pathology of the group of 18 patients who received triiodothyronine. For all these patients, the histological diagnosis of glioblastoma multiforme had been made before radiation and triiodothyronine were given. We were able to review the histology of 13 of the 18 patients. There were 18 specimens, 9 in the form of biopsy specimens and 9 as autopsy specimens. Eleven were astrocytoma grade IV and 5 were astrocytoma grade III. Two were equivocal grade III–IV. Of the 3 long-term survivors, 2 were grade III, those who survived 360 and 304 weeks, whereas the patient who survived for 352 weeks had astrocytoma grade IV.

DISCUSSION

Although the patients were not randomly assigned to different treatment groups, the observation does represent a sequential study in which all eligible patients during a period of 3 years were placed in the triiodothyronine study. The reason for using triiodothyronine as the radiosensitizing agent has been discussed by Griem and co-workers.[4, 5] Triiodothyronine may cause a metabolic change in tissue oxygenation at the cellular level; the increased blood flow to the tumor tissue and the resultant oxygenation could be the reason for the empiric observations made here. Also, triiodothyronine may recruit cells into the cell cycle; this in turn, would increase the number of cells susceptible to radiation. Griem and co-workers have demonstrated an increase in radiosensitivity of tissues when animals were treated by subcutaneous injection of triiodothyronine.[6] The effect of thyroid compound on the metabolic change of some organs and tissues is not uniformly equal. Chang and co-workers have shown that the radiosensitivity of patients with malignant gliomas increased when they were treated with hyperbaric oxygen and radiation therapy and have reported an increase in survival for this method of treatment.[2] Walker and co-workers have recently made a randomized control study on the efficacy of BCNU in conjunction with radiation therapy. The mean survival of the group of patients receiving BCUN and radiation was 41 weeks.[12]

The fact that tissue doses between 4000 and 4200 rads were used further suggests the increased radiosensitivity of this tumor in the induced hyperthyroid state. Further investigation is needed, however, to determine what is the optimum dose that will result in longer survival when triiodothyronine is used. Further work on the biology of triiodothyronine is also needed, as is a study of the mechanism by which it increases the radiosensitivity of these gliomas.

REFERENCES

1. Broder, L. Z., and Rall, D. P.: Chemotherapy of Brain Tumors. *Progr. Exptl. Tumor Res.* **17**:373–399 (1972).

2. Chang, C. H., Housepian, I. M., Sciarria, D., and Herbert, C. M.: Hyperbaric Oxygen and Radiation Therapy for Malignant Gliomas. In Seydel, H. G., Ed., *Tumors of the Nervous System.* Wiley, New York, 1974, p. 000.

3. Griem, M. L., Malkinson, F. D., and Morse, P. H.: Modification of Radiation Responses of Tissue by Colchicine. *Radiology* **77**:486–492 (1961).

4. Griem, M. L., and Stein, J. A.: Effect of Triiodothyronine on Radiosensitivity. *Nature* **182**:1681–1682 (1958).

5. Griem, M. L., and Stein, J. A.: The Effect of L-Triiodothyronine on Radiation Sensitivity. *Amer. J. Roentgen. Rad. Therapy., Nucl. Med.* **84**:695–698 (1960).

6. Griem, M. L., Stein, J. A., Reinertson, R. P., Reinertson, R., and Brown B. R.: Comparison of Effects of I^{131}-Induced Hyperthyroidism and L-Triiodothyronine on Irradiated Hair Roots in Mice. *Radiation Res.* **15**:202–210 (1961).

7. Jelsema, R., and Bucy, P. C.: Glioblastoma Multiforme: Its Treatment and Some Factors Affecting Survival. *Arch. Neurol.* **20**:161–171 (1969).

8. Jelsema, R., and Bucy, P. C.: The Treatment of Glioblastoma Multiforme of the Brain. *J. Neurosurg.* **27**:388–400 (1967).

9. Kernohen, J. W., and Sayre, G. P.: Tumors of the Central Nervous System. *A. F. I. P. Fascicle,* 1952.

10. Order, S. G., Hellman, S., Essen, C. F. von, and Kligerman, M. M.: Improvement in Quality of Survival Following Whole-Brain Irradiation for Brain Metastasis. *Radiology* **91**:149–153 (1968).

11. Suit, H. D.: Statement of the Problems Pertaining to the Effect of Dose Fractionation and Total Treatment Time on Response of Tissue to X-irradiation. *Conference on Time and Dose Relationship in Radiation Biology as Applied to Radiotherapy,* 1970, Upton, New York: Brookhaven National Laboratory, 1970, pp. vii–x.

12. Walker, M. D., and Gehan, G. A.: An Evaluation of BCNU and Irradiation Alone and in Combination for the Treatment of Malignant Glioma. Abstract presented at the National Conference on Cancer Chemotherapy, 1972.

13. Wilson, C. B., and Hoshino, T.: Current Trends in the Chemotherapy of Brain Tumors with Special Reference to Glioblastoma. *J. Neurosurg.* **31**:589–603 (1969).

Hyperbaric Oxygen and Radiation Therapy for Malignant Gliomas

Chu H. Chang, M.D.,

Professor of Radiology, College of Physicians and Surgeons,
Columbia University, New York, New York;
Director, Division of Radiotherapy,
Columbia-Presbyterian Medical Center,
New York, New York

Edgar M. Housepian, M.D.,

Associate Professor of Clinical Neurological Surgery,
College of Physicians and Surgeons,
Columbia University, New York, New York;
Associate Attending Neurological Surgeon, Neurological Institute,
Columbia-Presbyterian Medical Center, New York, New York

Daniel Sciarra, M.D.,

Professor of Clinical Neurology,
College of Physicians and Surgeons,
Columbia University, New York, New York;
Attending Neurologist, Neurological Institute,
Columbia-Presbyterian Medical Center,
New York, New York

Charles M. Herbert, Jr., A.B.,

Associate, College of Physicians and Surgeons,
Columbia University, New York, New York;
Radiation Physicist, Division of Radiotherapy,
Columbia-Presbyterian Medical Center,
New York, New York

M olecular oxygen has long been known as one of the most powerful dose-modi-
fying agents for the biological effect of x-radiation. In 1953 Gray[1] reported that
the biological effect of x-rays is increased by a factor of about 3 when x-irradiation is
performed under well-oxygenated condition as compared to anoxic conditions. This
oxygen effect has subsequently been confirmed in many mammalian tissue culture
systems and in experimental solid-tumor models. However, a significant improvement
in clinical results of radiotherapy of human cancer with hyperbaric oxygen is yet to be
established.

Malignant glioma is considered one of the unique tumors for the clinical trial of the
oxygen effect in radiotherapy because of the following: (1) Malignant glioma runs a
rapid and uniformly fatal course. Survival following neurosurgical decompression and
conventional radiotherapy can be measured in terms of months, a greater than 90%
mortality within 18 months, so that the treatment results can be assessed in a
reasonably short period of time. (2) A high incidence of necrosis and hemorrhage is
present in malignant glioma, whereby an anoxic or hypoxic tumor cell subpopulation
most likely exists. (3) Malignant glioma is confined in the cranial cavity and an extracranial metastases is an exceedingly rare occurrence, so that the tumor can be adequately encompassed in the irradiated volume without escape.

The available methods for restoring tissue oxygen tension in human tumors during
radiotherapy include: (1) breathing pure oxygen under increased atmospheric pressure
in a compression chamber;[2] (2) breathing oxygen and carbon dioxide (95% and 5%,
respectively) under atmospheric pressure through a nose mask;[3, 4] and (3) intraarterial
injection of hydrogen peroxide in the tumor region.[5]

Hyperbaric oxygenation appears to be highly efficient because by breathing oxygen
under high pressure (3–4 atm, absolute), the partial pressure of oxygen in the arterial
blood and the solubility of oxygen in physiologic solution may increase 20- to 30-fold.[6]

In 1963 we acquired a new transparent pressure chamber made of Lucite and manu-
factured by Vickers and Co. of London, England. The new chamber is operated at a
pressure of 3 atm (absolute). At this pressure, the frequency of convulsion due to
oxygen toxicity is greatly reduced and the need for general anesthesia is thus
eliminated. With the elimination of general anesthesia, many more fractionated treatments can be given to the patients than with the previous limited 2 or 3 massive dose[7]
treatments. However, with the increase of the number of fractions, reassessment of the
time–dose relationship and biologic response is necessary.

PATIENTS AND METHODS

At the Neurological Institute of Columbia-Presbyterian Medical Center, New York,
about 30 cases of malignant glioma are seen and treated per year, among which 15 are
tissue proven glioblastoma (or astrocytoma, grade III or IV). A pilot study[8] was set up
in late 1963, with an initial dose schedule of 3600 rads in 3 weeks, that is, 400 rads per
treatment, 3 treatments per week (TIW), in a total of 9 treatments, using a radiocobalt
source and bilateral opposing wide-field technique. This was a conservative dosage to
begin with, but we wanted to avoid the potential deleterious effect of combined oxygen
and radiation in unconventional fractionation. The dose was systematically increased to

This investigation was supported by Public Health Services Research Grant No. CA-07962 from
the National Cancer Institute.

4000 rads in 3⅓ weeks (400 rads, TIW); 4400 rads in 3⅔ weeks (400 rads, TIW), and 5000 rads in 5 weeks (333 rads, TIW), as our experience with the oxygen toxicity and brain tissue tolerance increased. Since 1969, the dosage and fractionation have been changed to 6000 rads in 6 weeks on a 5-treatments per week schedule; the initial 3000 rads are delivered to the whole brain and the subsequent 3000 rads to a reduced volume encompassing the demonstrable tumor volume. This pilot study was designed to include eventually a pair-arrangement technique whereby one in the pair was treated with pure oxygen breathing under 3 atm pressure (30 psi) and the other without oxygen as a control. This technique was followed as closely as possible, but was not in strictly random fashion due to the initial difficult clinical situation.

Treatment Procedure

The treatment is usually commenced on the day when the scalp wound sutures are removed. Bilateral myringotomies are usually done 1 day before the course of radio-therapy. A premedication with a sedative (such as Seconal 100 mg IM) is given half an hour prior to going into the pressure chamber. The head is immobilized with a special tape holder and the localization port film is obtained. The chamber (Fig. 1) is then flushed at atmospheric pressure with 100% oxygen until 90% oxygen content in the chamber is obtained. The pressurization is then begun until 30 psi is reached (3 atm absolute). The pressurization usually takes 5–6 minutes. At this time the oxygen concentration in the chamber is measured and is usually 99+%, as indicated by a Beckman model D oxygen analyzer. The pressure is maintained at this level for 15 minutes for adequate oxygen diffusion outside cerebral capillaries before the irradiation

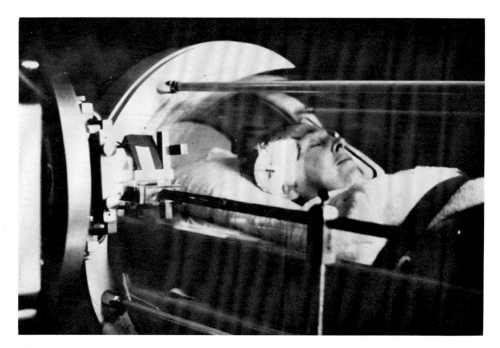

Fig. 1. A transparent high-pressure oxygen chamber made of lucite cylinders (Vickers Limited, London, England) 7 ft long and 2 ft internal diameter.

is given. The decompression begins as soon as irradiation is over and takes about 3–4 minutes. The control group is irradiated without the pressure chamber in normal atmospheric air, with the same dose fractionation as in the study group.

RESULTS

There were 83 patients admitted to the project, 41 patients with hyperbaric oxygen and 42 as control. Two early patients in the oxygen group are excluded because the oxygen treatment was given for recurrent glioblastomas several months after the initial course of radiotherapy (Table 1).

Survival Rate

An acturial method of analysis is applied and the survival rate is depicted in two curves (Fig. 2). Curve A shows the survival rate of the oxygen group (surgery, radiotherapy and oxygen) and curve B shows that of control group (surgery and radiotherapy). Curve A shows a slightly higher survival rate at 3-month intervals for the oxygen group than for the control group. The average 50% survival rate is about 2 months longer in the oxygen group than in the control group. At the end of 18 months the survival rate for the oxygen group is about 22% and for the control group about 9%. At 24 months, both curves tend to converge at a lower survival level. By the end of 30 months, these two curves appear to merge. However, we still have 3 survivors in the oxygen group who are alive at 18, 17, and 15 months and 1 survivor in the control group alive beyond 15 months so that the shape of the later portions of these two curves cannot be predicted at this time. Because of small population samples, a preliminary evaluation employing exact probabilities was used to screen the data for possible statistical signifi-

TABLE 1. GLIOBLASTOMA (GRADES III AND IV): CASE DISTRIBUTION IN CLINICAL TRIAL, OXYGEN STUDY GROUP VS AIR CONTROL

Fractionation Scheme	No. of Cases in Each Trial Group	
	Oxygen Study Group (OHP at 30 psi)	Air Control Group
3600 rads/3 weeks (400 rad, TIW) NSD = 1540 ret	9	10
4000 rads/3½ weeks (400 rad, TIW) NSD = 1650 ret	4	4
4400 rads/3⅔ weeks (400 rad, TIW) NSD = 1750 ret	2	6
5000 rads/5 weeks (333 rad, TIW) NSD = 1780 ret	6	7
6000 rads/6 weeks (200 rad QD) NSD = 1770 ret	18	15
Total	39	42

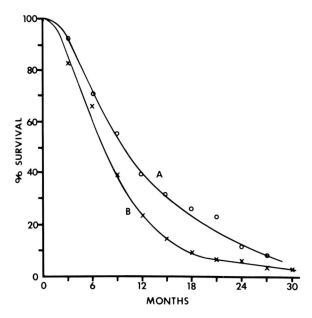

Fig. 2. Survival curves of glioblastoma (astrocytoma grade III and IV): (*A*) radiotherapy and hyperbaric oxygen study group; (*B*) radiotherapy air control group.

cance. The results indicate that no statistically significant difference exists between the two groups.

Quality of Survival

Those who completed a course of radiotherapy under hyperbaric oxygen seemed to enjoy a better quality of survival than the radiotherapy control group. For example, 1 patient who was a manager of a supermarket was able to return to his job in full capacity for at least 6 months following a course of radiotherapy under hyperbaric oxygen. Another patient who was a banker, returned to work for 1 year before he was advised to retire.

Complications

Most patients tolerated the hyperbaric oxygen procedure well. Some of them continued their treatments as out-patients after having received initial treatments for 1 or 2 weeks in the hospital. Only 2 patients developed generalized convulsion at the time of decompression due to oxygen toxicity. The incidence is less than $\frac{1}{2}\%$ in terms of the total number of exposures in our series. Several patients developed mild otitis media following myringotomy and hyperbaric therapy. One patient developed severe skin reaction with subsequent disruption of scalp wound. Three patients had extensive radiation necrosis of the brain observed at a subsequent "second look" surgery or at autopsy.

DISCUSSION

This preliminary report represents a prospective clinical study of pilot nature. We have not accomplished a strict randomization in this series of patients.

During the course of this study, we have observed microscopically that a glioblastoma could be completely destroyed by irradiation under hyperbaric oxygen, probably in the dose level of 4000 rads in $3\frac{1}{3}$ weeks and above in 3 treatments per week schedule (NSD = 1650 ret). The autopsy material of 1 patient with glioblastoma showed a complete disappearance of tumor cells in the irradiated postoperative tumor field. However, the radionecrosis of the normal brain tissue appeared to be extensive.

On the other hand, we have also observed actively growing recurrent tumor nodules in the previously irradiated field in a few patients who had clinical recurrence of glioblastoma and who subsequently received a "second-look" operation.

Glioblastoma is one of the most malignant and rapidly fatal tumors. A 5-year survivor of glioblastoma is an exception rather than a rule. There is a possibility that the initial diagnosis of the 5-year survivors was incorrect, either because of misinterpretation or missampling of a lower grade astrocytoma of grade II as grade III or because of the presence of a slow-growing variant of the tumor.

For assessment of the response of glioblastoma to a new treatment technique, it has been our policy to start with a dosage system working from the lower dose range upward instead of from the higher range downward so that any untoward normal tissue damage can be detected early and the technique modified. In the dose system we used in this study, we encountered few untoward reactions until 4400 rads in $3\frac{1}{3}$ weeks with 400 rads per treatment and 3 treatments per week was reached. At present, we use a schedule of 6000 rads in 6 weeks (200 rads per treatment and 5 treatments per week). The initial 3000 rads are given in air and the subsequent 3000 rads under hyperbaric oxygenation. The rational is based on recent radiobiological evidence that reoxygenation of hypoxic tumor cells takes place soon after conventional daily irradiation. It is conceivable that only residual hypoxic tumor cells in the core of the tumor would require hyperbaric oxygen to enhance their killing in the last part of the course of radiotherapy. It has been noted[9] that it is the size of the dose per fraction rather than the number of fractions that accounts more for the degree of radiation injury of the normal brain tissues. Under the present clinical trial conditions, including a varying fractionation scheme and tumor dose level and a constant oxygen tension applied, it appears that there is no striking improvement of the survival rate over that with conventional irradiation. There are several other centers[10-12] that have also been engaged in the study of the effect of hyperbaric oxygen in radiotherapy of glioblastoma at one time or another.

SUMMARY

A pilot clinical trial on radiotherapy of glioblastoma with and without hyperbaric oxygen has been carried out at the Columbia-Presbyterian Medical Center. Eighty three cases of postoperative tissue proven glioblastoma have been admitted to the study, 41 were irradiated under hyperbaric oxygenation and 42 in atmospheric air as a control.

The survival rates for those previously untreated patients, 39 in the oxygen group and 42 in the control were evaluated by the acturial analysis method. Although the average 50% survival is about 2 months longer in the oxygen group than the control group, and at the end of 18 months, the survival rate is slightly higher in the oxygen group (22%) than the control group (9%), a preliminary statistical evaluation indicates that there is no significant difference in survival rates between the two groups.

The hyperbaric oxygen procedure is well tolerated by most patients. The quality of survival in the hyperbaric oxygen group appears to be equal or slightly better than that of the control group.

REFERENCES

1. Gray, L. H., Conger, A. D. Ebert, M., Hornsey, S., and Scott, O. C. A.: The Concentration of Oxygen Dissolved in Tissues at the Time of Irradiation as a Factor in Radiotherapy. *Brit. J. Radiol.* **26:**638 (1953).

2. Churchill-Davidson, I., Sanger, C., and Thomlinson, R. H.: High Pressure Oxygen and Radiotherapy. *Lancet* **1955-I:**1091.

3. DuSault, L. A.: Effect of Oxygen in Response of Spontaneous Tumor in Mice to Radiotherapy. *Brit. J. Radiol.* **36:**749–754 (1963).

4. Evans, J. C., and Sanfillippo, L. J.: Oxygen Tension of Oral Cavity Carcinoma. *Radiol. Clin. Biol.,* **39:**54–58 (1970).

5. Mallams, J. T., Balla, G. A., and Finney, J. W.: Regional Oxygenation and Radiation Therapy: Current Status. *Amer. J. Roentgenol. Rad. Therapy Nucl. Med.* **93:**160–169 (1965).

6. Lamphier, E. H.: Determinants of Oxygenation. In Clinical Application of Hyperbaric Oxygenation. Boerema, I., Ed., Elsevier, Amsterdam, 1964, pp. 277–283.

7. Atkins, H. L., Seaman, W. B., Jacox, H. W., and Matteo, R. S.: Experience with Hyperbaric Oxygenation in Clinical Radiotherapy. *Amer. J. Roentgenol. Rad. Therapy Nucl. Med.* **93:**651–663 (1965).

8. Chang, C. H., Seaman, W. B., and Jacox, H. W.: Clinical Aspects of Hyperbaric Oxygen and Radiotherapy: New York Experience. *Frontiers Rad. Therapy Oncol.* **1:**183–188 (1968).

9. Chang, C. H., Herbert, C., Jr., and Mastri, A.: Modification of Delayed Radiation Damage of Normal Brain Tissue in Cats by Hyperbaric Oxygenation and Dose Fractionation. In preparation.

10. Churchill-Davidson, I.: Hyperbaric Oxygen and Radiotherapy. Clinical Experiences. *Frontiers Radiation Therapy Oncol.* **1:**156–161 (1968).

11. Van Den Brenk, H. A. S., Madigan, J. P., and Kerr, R. C.: Experience with Megavoltage Irradiation of Advanced Malignant Disease Using High Pressure Oxygen. In Clinical Application of Hyperbaric Oxygenation. Boerema, I., Ed., Elsevier, Amsterdam, 1964, pp. 144–160.

12. Kramer, S.: Personal communication, 1971.

Discussion

Dr. Seydel. Dr. Griem, if you look at the figures there seems to have been a difference in thyroid status and a difference in age. How much does the age have to do with increased survival?

Dr. Griem. I don't know how one solves this problem of age. Certainly as the patient gets older the probability of his dying from automobile accidents, cardiac problems, and so forth is high and I think that certainly affects any series. Certainly in our series the patients that were made hyperthyroid were younger. So I don't have any answer to that. I think the way to do this is what we planned to do, and that is to start out and do a proper randomized trial now and see if this whole thing holds up. As far as the grading of the tumors is concerned, we didn't find any significant number of grade III, the bulk of them were grade IV.

We have two nice animal models, one is a chemically induced brain tumor which looks promising and which occurs in a rat, and we have a virus-induced brain tumor in the rat and the dog, and I think if one is able to produce 50 rat tumors and dog tumors and they are all alike, why then are you able to come up with answers much quicker. Now the two virus-induced tumors are both RNA-virus-induced tumors. The newborn animal is injected and if you inject it properly you get gliomas. The second thing is that these animals come down with the tumor in about 3 weeks and are dead in about 4 weeks, so the answers come up rather rapidly and I think that before we go back to doing a large series of patients we will do the dog work.

Discussant. Are you treating any patients currently?

Dr. Griem. We are trying high-grade gliomas in children to start out a randomized trial. Here again is another area where the results are not very favorable. Now the children incidentally tolerate the hyperthyroid stage very nicely as out-patients and we can get their BMRs up plus 20, the pulses run 120, 130 and they seem to handle this as out-patients.

Dr. Seydel. I should like to ask Dr. Mullan what the age has to do with the survival of patients with gliomas?

Dr. Mullan. I think this is an extraordinarily important factor. There are glioblastomas and glioblastomas and the pathologist looks at the slide and he says this a gliobastoma grade IV, and half a dozen pathologists look at the slide and they all say it's glioblastoma grade IV, but you and I and everyone who is in the clinical aspect know that these may be entirely different. For example, I think a glioblastoma in a man aged 60 is entirely different from a glioblastoma in a younger person. So I think sticking strictly to histological category we will fall into pitfalls unless we take the complete clinical presentation of the patient as well and here I think the age factor is a very very important one.

Dr. Seydel. Dr. Kramer, would you like to comment regarding gliomas, age and survival?

Dr. Kramer. I quite agree with Dr. Mullan but I think there is also a question of the general condition of the patient. I think it's a clinical impression that we have and I don't have any good data on that although there ought to be that often times we see a younger patient with very much better general condition although the histological grade is III or IV, and therefore the patient would stand a better chance of survival. I think the thing has been pointed as one of the most difficult problems. And that is the histological stratification of these patients. We all appreciate the difficulties the pathologist has because often he is given a relatively small portion of tissue and we all know that these tumors vary a great deal between one portion of the tumor and another. It's one thing to look at the thing in a postmortem specimen where you can survey the whole situation or when you have to make a decision on a relatively small specimen. It's also unfortunate I think that there is still such a great variation in classification. There are some people who adamantly refuse to grade their tumors into I through IV and they lump all the malignant tumors together into the glioblastoma group, whereas others do stratify and I think that there is some point in the stratification that is borne out both by the figures shown from the Mayo Clinic where the grade III's survived far better than the grade IV's and in our own experience where we have some 5 out of 25 grade III's alive at 5 years and 0 out of 75 grade IV's. So there is a need for this classification but there is a large gap it seems to me between the need and how it is going to be done. And I think this may be one of the difficulties in Dr. Griem's series that you obviously will not be able to render hyperthyroid the very ill patients. Regarding oxygenation of the tumor in the hyperbaric chamber, there are tremendous difficulties. It seems very sensible that if you can increase the oxygenation of the tumor you are going to get better results, but we don't really know that putting a patient into the hyperbaric tank increases the oxygenation of the tumor cells. I think this is one of the great difficulties, and we must congratulate Dr. Chang on this tremendous effort because to put that number of patients through hyperbaric oxygenation and irradiation is an enormous effort and one again has to think in terms of a cost effectiveness. This is a very long run for a very short slide.

Discussant.   I have heard a couple of excellent papers on the effects of hyperthermia both as a direct antitumor effect and also as a radiation sensitizer. I wanted to ask Dr. Griem if he thinks that the raising of the body temperature with these high doses of T_3 is a significant factor. What I am asking is: Is hyperthermia part of the response, perhaps separate from the effects of oxygenation?

Dr. Griem.   All of these patients were hospitalized and we didn't know that the temperature charts indicated that they had fever during the treatment. I don't think that plays a role. We tried induced hyperthermia in patients in 1962 after it was suggested that this might be a way of increasing the radiosensitivity. This can be produced with the use of etiocholanalone which is a metabolic steroid. Regular fever can be produced about 1 hour after starting the intravenous drip with this material without all the problems of other methods of producing fever. Unfortunately we did not induce hyperthermia in any brain-tumor patients.

Dr. Kjellberg.   Just one comment while we are on gliomas. My talk this afternoon is about protons but we are using some protons on glioma patients in a combined proton–photon technique where the patient gets a full course of x-ray to about 4500 rads and then protons to the defined tumor volume as defined by angiography or scanning. We seek to deliver an incremental dose to produce necrosis within that volume. We have a few good cases but I don't believe that we could stand any kind of statistical challenge.

Discussant. Dr. Griem, have you had any experience or do you have any data on using T_3 enhancement of chemotherapeutic agents, particularly radiomimetic agents such as actinomycin D or cytoxan?

Dr. Griem. I believe someone mixed nitrogen mustard and T_3 together around '63 and found some enhancement. I think it is an interesting question. One has really to go back to the drawing board. I think it's time to quit the mixing of this and that together and I think one needs to go to cell cultures or tumor models and to look at growth fractions. If you can put more cells into the mitotic cycle then you are capable of using cycle-linked chemotherapeutic agents like vincristine or hydroxyurea. There is a whole host of cycle-linked chemotherapeutic agents, whereas nitrogen mustard and alkalating agents are not cycled. The reason that some of the combination chemotherapeutic agents work is that, for example, DeVita and Carbone have looked at these questions and have come up with logical combinations that work on proper areas of the cell cycle. And it may be that thyroid or other agents will recruit cells into cycle will be important in future chemotherapy.

Dr. Jones. I would like to ask Dr. Chang and Dr. Kramer to comment on multicentric disease in glioblastoma and its relationship to oxygen tension.

Dr. Chang. Multicentric involvement of the glioblastoma is not too common. In autopsy material we rarely obtained typical multicentric tumor because most patients show diffusely infiltrative involvement. Real multicentric tumor probably occurs in less than 10%. In that case I think whole brain irradiation certainly would be indicated, but I still don't have a firm figure to tell you.

Dr. Kramer. We really know very little about oxygen tension both in the brain and in brain tumors. There is some evidence that we have a good deal more hypoxia in a normal brain than we care to admit and more than we know about, and if that is true then, of course, the use of high LET radiation may be disastrous rather than effective because you lower the oxygen enhancement ratio both for normal tissue and for brain tumor. Perhaps one of the reasons we have got away with relatively high doses is that the normal brain is somewhat hypoxic, but we just don't know enough about it, I think. As for multicentric gliomas, I think in most cases if you dissect them carefully you will find a connection even in those patients that appear to have two separate gliomas. I think the only diffuse situation I can think of perhaps is the gliomatous meningitis. In rare patients the glioma diffusely invades the surface of the brain. In my experience these patients have done rather poorly.

Dr. Munzenrider. I would like to ask Dr. Griem if he had any patients with glioblastomas treated with the T_3 alone.

Dr. Griem. No. When rats were treated with T_3 the tumors grew wildly and one could actually see these tumors grow day by day. When compared with the other rats who were given T_3 and radiation there was quite a difference, and we felt that we did not want to do that arm of the protocol at that time.

Chemotherapy of Brain Tumors of Childhood

W. A. Newton, Jr., M.D.,
Professor of Pathology and Pediatrics,
Ohio State University,
Children's Hospital, Columbus Ohio

Inta J. Ertel, M.D.,
Associate Professor of Pediatrics,
Ohio State University,
Children's Hospital,
Columbus, Ohio

Janak Wadwa, M.D.,
Clinical Assistant
   Professor of Pediatrics,
Ohio State University,
Children's Hospital,
Columbus, Ohio

M. P. Sayers, M.D.,
Associate Professor of the
Department of Surgery,
Division of Neurosurgery,
Ohio State University;
Chief of Neurosurgery,
Children's Hospital,
Columbus, Ohio

Despite modernization and improved techniques in surgery and intensification of efforts in radiotherapy of brain tumors in children, the prognosis of the majority of types of brain cancer in childhood is poor particularly in those involving the brain stem, medulloblastomas, and ependymomas, all common tumors of childhood. For this reason the possible adjunctive use of chemotherapy should be seriously considered, especially since chemotherapy has significantly altered survival in a number of childhood tumors including Wilms' tumor and rhabdomyosarcoma.

In the initial phases of the use of drugs to treat cancer, compounds were given to patients with a variety of tumors in an attempt to evaluate the possible effectiveness of a given compound. As a rule chemotherapy was initially given to patients who had recurrent disease or metastatic tumor rather than early in the course of therapy. While palliation was possible utilizing drugs late in the course of the cancer in the patient, it has been subsequently shown that an increased cure rate cannot be accomplished by drugs at that late time, but depends on drugs given early in the course of the disease at the time when potential cancer residual is subclinical. It has been demonstrated that clinical cancer diagnosis is dependent on the presence of an arbitrary number of cancer cells somewhere in the range of 10^{12}. Drugs given to patients with this amount of tumor have not effected cures. It is only when a sizable amount of tumor is removed or when it is reduced in size or eliminated by the use of radiation therapy that chemotherapy has been able to significantly affect the course of the disease. Patients with localized Wilms' tumor, after removal of their primary lesion still had approximately 55% pulmonary metastatic rate. However, when prophylactic chemotherapy is given following radiation therapy and initial surgery, an addition 30% of the patients can be salvaged.

Likewise, patients with rhabdomyosarcoma treated with repeated courses of drugs following surgery and/or radiation have shown a marked increase in their survival rate from approximately 10% to somewhere around 70% when the lesions are localized at diagnosis. The optimum use of chemotherapy would therefore appear to be (*1*) for the tumor that is responsive to chemotherapy and (*2*) at a time when the residual tumor cell population is at a minimum.

The use of cancer chemotherapy has been perhaps slowest in the area of the treatment of brain tumors for a number of reasons.[1] Early there was a lack of a suitable animal model to test the compounds. Several models have recently been developed that have enabled investigators to obtain preliminary data that can be applied to patients. Secondly, there has been a lack of reliable means of drug selection for individual tumors like those indications afforded by effectiveness of the given compound in childhood leukemia or acute leukemia. Thirdly, there is a lack of a rapid system for precise measurement of tumor response and for the most part on the clinician's judgement must be relied upon for short-term changes and survival, a measurement that consumes considerable time. Development of techniques such as scintillation brain scanning has afforded additional refinement, but there still is an imprecise measurement of response. In addition, the drugs commonly used for cancer are given either orally or parenterally. The blood–brain barrier presents a unique problem when compounds of the usual variety are given in their customary fashion.

Chemotherapy of CNS disease with cancer chemotherapy agents is not new since

This study was supported in part by the National Institutes of Health Research Grant No. 2 R10 CA 03750.

intrethecal administration of methotrexate has been used for the treatment of meningeal leukemia for many years. Because of the effectiveness of ITMTX in meningeal leukemia, Dr. Sayers and our staff attempted to use this drug in this route to evaluate the possible beneficial effects in a variety of children's tumors. In a summary prepared several years ago[2] 44 children (who had a variety of malignant brain tumors including astrocytoma, medulloblastoma, and ependymoma) were given 1–5 courses of methotrexate in a dose of 0.25 mg/kg intrethecally for 5–7 daily doses. Nineteen children were given this type of therapy alone after conventional therapy had been given and this treatment could be thus evaluated as a single parameter of therapy. Objective neurologic findings were shown to improve and be alleviated in 15 of 19 patients; others obtained transitory subjective relief. Periods of improvement tended to be relatively brief, however, lasting to 1½–5 months in most patients. Toxic reactions were minimal and reversible with the exception of 1 patient who developed a severe bone marrow depression when the methotrexate was given concurrently with parenteral chloramphenicol for sepsis. It was pointed out at that time that while this was essentially a potential approach, that application of this type of medication or others should be tried earlier in the disease prior to evidences of clinical recurrence. While this has been tried in a few patients, sufficient data has not been obtained to draw any conclusions.

Several authors reported responses to a variety of childhood brain tumors to intravenous vincristine.[3-8] This has been common experience since then and has now become an established form of palliative therapy in a variety of childhood brain tumors.

The Brain Tumor Study Group has been active in studying the effect of a variety of drugs in adult brain tumors beginning with mithramycin for advanced glioblastoma multiforme. Results of these studies were not startling, but led this group to continue their investigations.[9, 10]

Recently Walker and Gehan reported an encouraging result in the evaluation of BCNU,[11] a nitrosourea compound. A prospective controlled randomized study was carried out in which adult patients with malignant gliomas were given BCNU in addition to radiation and the results were compared to a similar group treated with radiation alone. All patients received conventional neurosurgical care including tumor resection with adequate decompression. The histologic diagnosis confirmed a malignant glioma. The preliminary analysis of 180 patients showed the control survival times of 17 weeks, BCNU 20 weeks, radiation alone 28 weeks, and BCNU plus radiation 41 weeks, a significant change with a p value of less than .01.

When combined with vincristine, BCNU was not quite as effective as the drug itself when tried in the 81 patients with recurrent primary or metastatic brain tumors as reported by Fewer et al in 1972.[12] An analog of this compound, CCNU, likewise a nitrosourea, has also shown effects on recurrent malignant brain tumors, and ethyl CCNU has been reported to have similar effects by Young et al in 1973.[13]

The following is a summary of the experiences at Children's Hospital, Columbus, Ohio, utilizing chemotherapy for brain tumors over the past 5 years. These are patients who were given therapy during this period rather than diagnosed during this period. There were a total of 24 of 115 new patients who were given therapy with drugs as a part of their management. The sites of their tumors include 5 with origin in the ventricular systems, 6 in the brain stem, 2 supratentorial lesions, 7 cerebellar tumors, 1 of the optic chiasm, 1 of the hypothalamus, 1 meningeal infiltration, and 1 is a benign tumor of choroid plexus. The diagnoses include 5 with ependymomas, 4 medulloblastomas, and 6 astrocytomas, and 6 had no tissue diagnosis. The drugs were given to 22 of the 24 for recurrence of tumor or for active disease; 2 were given in the absence of disease prophylactically. The drugs included methotrexate given intrathecally, vincristine given intravenously, CCNU given orally, and cytoxan given intrathecally. Some received only one drug. Others received several, usually in sequence. Intrathecal methotrexate (ITMTX) was used alone in 10 instances, vincristine (VCR), CCNU, and cytoxan alone in 1 each. Intrathecal methotrexate, vincristine, and CCNU were used in 6 patients.

The results of therapy are as follows: Of this group of patients, there are 6 still living, but 18 have expired. Two patients are living without tumor, 2 are known to have tumor, and in 2 others it is not certain whether or not tumor exists at the present time. The 2 known not to have tumor include 1 patient surviving 28 months who had repeated courses of intrathecal methotrexate given prophylactically, and a second patient who has received a series of 4 courses of CCNU and is surviving 9 months. The 2 patients with tumor include 1 surviving 15 months with thalamic glioma, and 1 living 4½ years with occipital astrocytoma. Of those with questionable residual tumor, 1 patient is living 5 years with a previously treated astrocytoma of the cerebellum and 1 patient is living 6 years after being diagnosed as having medulloblastoma. This latter patient was treated with 5 courses of intrathecal methotrexate but this was not given prophylactically in the absence of disease.

The clinical response to chemotherapy in these patients is as follows: Of 9 patients receiving ITMTX, 4 showed both objective and subjective response, 2 subjective only, and 1 no response; 1 received prophylactic therapy only, and treatment effects could not be evaluated in another. Six of 10 receiving vincristine showed both objective and subjective response, but no response was seen in 4. Five of 8 receiving CCNU achieved both objective and subjective response, 1 had no response, and 2 could not be evaluated. Fourteen patients received inadequate amount of drug to evaluate.

Our latest study is designed to utilize our three most effective drugs, ITMTX, CCNU, and VCR, in a repetative cycle following initial surgery and radiation for a period of 1 year. Thus far 3 patients have been placed on this regimen for periods of 20, 13, and 12 weeks.

The following is the case of a patient who has received CCNU chemotherapy, with demonstration of reduction in tumor size following chemotherapy alone. A. T. was diagnosed as having a hypothalamic tumor at the age of 5 years, histologically astrocytoma grade II. He received 5000 rads to the tumor mass from December 7, 1972 to January 26, 1973. In April of 1973, he developed increased clumsiness, decreased visual acuity, and pallor of his fundi. A brain scan done at the time of diagnosis showed a 5-cm mass. In April the tumor still was present (Fig. 1), so the child was started on CCNU 130 mg/m² every 6 weeks. He became more active and asymptomatic. A repeat brain scan done on September 5 showed virtual absence of demonstrable increased uptake in the area where the tumor had previously been found (Fig. 2).

We have been informed that in a study carried out during 1970 and 1971 children with brain tumors at the Institute Gustave-Roussy in France[14] were given conventional surgery and radiation therapy, and, in addition, prophylactic chemotherapy. The latter consisted of intrethecal methotrexate 0.04 mg/kg twice a week for 10 doses during the 5 weeks of radiation therapy. In the ninth week there was a repetitive cycle of IV vincristine for 6 doses, then a rest of 4 weeks, then 5 weeks of intramuscular methotrexate 0.75 mg/kg twice a week for 4 cycles. The results of this study showed that there

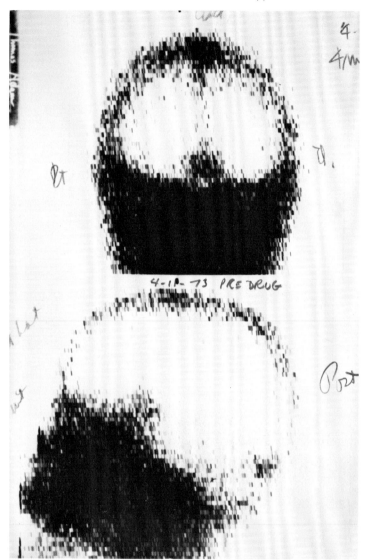

Fig. 1. ^{99m}Tc anterior and right lateral rectilinear scan on April 12, 1973, demonstrating a 3 cm third ventricular-hypothalamic lesion.

was no statistical difference in the survival rate or the duration of survival in this group of patients compared to those of similar nature in 1965 and 1969. A revision of the chemotherapy was instituted for 1972–1973, in which vincristine was given during the radiation in 4–6 weekly injections followed by a combination of vincristine and CCNU in the maintenance course. The results of this are not yet available. A current pilot study of radiotherapy and chemotherapy for medulloblastoma and ependymoma is being carried out at the Royal Marsden Hospital in which a combination of intrethecal methotrexate, vincristine and CCNU is used.[14]

Experimental studies have been carried out in recent years in an attempt to define the problems involved and to allow a mechanism for study of these problems. Several

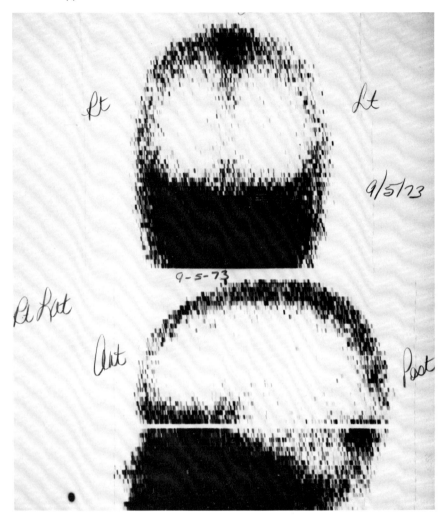

Fig. 2. ^{99m}Tc anterior and right lateral projections of rectilinear scans taken on September 5, 1973, showing minimal to absent activity in previously demonstrated tumor area of April 12, 1973.

animal tumor models have been developed including an ependymoblastoma mouse model that incorporates a readily transplantable tumor in small animals and makes it possible to reproduce brain tumors in large numbers of animals for statistically valid testing. Also four chemically induced lines of murine glioma have been used. A number of compounds have been evaluated utilizing these tumor systems where animal duration of survival is evaluated using the standard control test animals. Thus far the drugs for the best prolongation of survival have been nitrosoureas, CCNU and BCNU.

In addition, a number of studies have been carried out in an attempt to understand the dynamics of the localization of antitumor drugs in the tumor tissue in the brain and also their distribution in the brain itself. The relevance of these studies as a predictive human response has yet to be evaluated. The data derived from the isotope-labeled uptake experiments tend to confirm that the blood–brain barrier is not a significant impediment to entry of chemotherapeutic agents into the midst of brain tumors. It would appear that the blood vessels within the center of a brain tumor resemble vessels found outside the brain and are quite porous. It has been demonstrated, however, that while most of the cells in the brain tumor are located in the central regions, the actively proliferating cells are found along the edge. It is in such a site that the water-soluble drugs, including methotrexate, have restricted entry, while the lipid-soluble nitrosoureas may easily enter. Theoretically then the nitrosoureas are more effective because they can affect both cells in the center and the peripheral tumors.

Clearly there is considerable information to encourage the investigator to pursue studies in evaluation of chemotherapy compounds in treatment of childhood brain tumors. At present palliation certainly is real utilizing compounds that have already been shown to be effective, particularly intrethecal methotrexate, intravenous vincristine, and the nitrosoureas. The prophylactic use of drugs early in the therapy of the patient has yet to be adequately evaluated and may afford a significant change in the survival pattern of these serious lesions.

REFERENCES

1. Shapiro, W. R.: Malignant Brain Tumor Chemotherapy: Part 1 Experimental Studies. *Clin. Bull., Meorial Sloan-Kettering Cancer Center* 3:58–62 (1973).

2. Newton, W. A., Jr., Sayers, M. P., and Samuels, L. D.: Intrathecal Methotrexate (NSC-740) Therapy For Brain Tumors in Children. *Cancer Chemotherapy Rept.,* **52:**257 (1968).

3. Owens, G., Javid, R., Tallon, M., Stepanian, G., and Belmusto, L.: Arterial Infusion Chemotherapy of Primary Gliomas. *J. Amer. Med. Assoc.,* **186:**142 (1963).

4. Lassman, L. P., Pearce, G. W., and Gant, J.: Sensitivity of Intracranial Gliomas to Vincristine Sulphate. Lancet **1965-**296–297.

5. Owens, G., Javid, R., Belmusto, L., Bender, M., and Blau, M.: Intraarterial Vincristine Therapy of Primary Gliomas. *Cancer* **18(6):**756 (1965).

6. Lassman, L. P., Pearce, G. W., and Gang, J.: Effect of Vincristine Sylphate on the Intracranial Gliomata of Childhood. *Brit. J. Surg.* **53:**774 (June 1966).

7. Lampkin, B. C., Mauer, A. M., and McCride, B. H.: Response of Medulloblastoma to Vincristine Sulfate: A Case Report. *Pediatrics* **39:**761 (1967).

8. Smart, C. R., Ottoman, R. E., Rochlin, D. B., Harnes, J., Silva, A., and Goepfert, H.: Clinical Experience with Vincristine (NSC-67574) in Tumors of the Central Nervous System and other Malignant Diseases. *Cancer Chemotherapy Rept.,* **52:**733 (1968).

9. Kennedy, B. J., Brown, J. H., and Yarbro, J. W.: Mithramycin (NSC-24559) Therapy for Primary Glioblastomas. *Cancer Chemotherapy Rept.,* **48:**59–63, (October 1965).

10. Ransohoff, J., Martin, B. F., Medrek, T. J., Harris, M. N., Golomb, F. M., and Wright, J. C.: Preliminary Clinical Study of Mithramycin (NSC-24559) in Primary Tumors of the Central Nervous System. *Cancer Chemotherapy Rept.* **49:**51–57 (December 1965).

11. Walker, M. D., and Gehan, E. A.: An Evaluation of 1-3-BIS(2-Chlorethyl)-1-Nitrosourea (BCNU) and Irradiation Alone and in Combination for the Treatment of Malignant Glioma. *Proc. Amer. Assoc. Cancer Res.* **13:**67 (1972).

12. Fewer, D., Wilson, C. B., Boldrey, E. B., Enot, K. J., and Powell, M. R.: The Chemotherapy of Brain Tumors: Clinical Experience With Carmustine (BCNU) and Vincristine. *J. Amer. Med. Assoc.,* **222:**549, (Oct. 1972).

13. Young, R. C., Walker, M. D., Canellos, G. P., Schein, P. S., Chabner, B. A., and DeVita, W. T.: Initial Clinical Trials with Methyl-CCNU 1-(2-Chloroethyl)-3-(4-Methyl Cyclohexyl)-1-Nitrosourea (MeCCNU). *Cancer* **31:**1164 (1973).

14. Personal communication.

Discussion

Dr. Seydel. We have heard that radiotherapy and surgery form the basis of our present management but that chemotherapy provides additional therapy. Dr. Kramer would you like to comment regarding this please?

Dr. Kramer. I think this a very interesting presentation and I think we ought to try and establish sensitive ground rules. We are dealing with children's tumors. We are really not too concerned with prolonging life for a matter of months. I know that almost anything we do in the management of cancer is marginal advance but we must really try and look at the situation from the long-term survival. We are interested in 20 or 30 or 40 years or 50 years, not a few months. I think a very significant point is that most of the children's tumors we see in the brain are amenable to treatment and to long-term survival by radiation therapy. You take for instance the medulloblastoma, it's pretty well established now that we can with adequate treatment look to a 5-year survival rate of about 40% and a 10-year survival rate of 30%. I think this is well established in the literature now, and it's the same in our own group. But this means, of course, that ultimately about 70% of these patients will die of their tumors and it's an enormously important situation to try and do something for these patients. Now why do these patients die? In our experience most of them die of local recurrence in the cerebellum. A few die because of distant metastasis and we certainly see the metastasis in the neural axis but almost always with local recurrence in the cerebellum as well. Incidentally, most of the recurrences take place within the first 2 years after treatment and they become much less common after that. Therefore it seems to me enormously important to try and set up a trial to see whether the drugs that Dr. Newton has suggested, or any other drugs given in a persistent intermittent manner after the initial treatment, will prolong life. There really has not been a prospective trial and I think it is essential that such a prospective trial be set up for these patients in order to measure both the advantage and the possible disadvantage in such a trial. All we can say at the present moment is that the advance that chemotherapy has offered up until now has been relatively marginal even in the adults and that a clinical trial is urgently needed both as continuation of the clinical trials in the brain tumor study group and by setting up trials in childhood gliomas and medulloblastomas. I believe this is most important.

Dr. Seydel. I should like to ask Dr. Newton to comment regarding this. I also would like to ask him to comment regarding the quality of survival of these children. We all have seen children who have their tumors arrested or cured but who are mentally defective depending upon how you look at things.

Dr. Newton. Dr. Kramer, if you had given your remarks prior to my paper I would not have said anything. That is really what I said in effect, that we really are in the early stages. I believe in the application of chemotherapy. Whether or not it will eventually be as successful in this area as in other areas of the body in children is an important point. I think this is the important thing that the chemotherapy never will work successfully when we deal with end-stage disease and it has to be done in a prospective fashion. I could not agree more that we have to be very careful about the type of treatment we give people. All I can say is that at this point and time with brain tumors there is no question in my mind that we make life better for a longer period of time having used these drugs in the patients that I have been associated with in many instances. It is true that these patients are only palliated; but we go from a child who was incapacitated, slumped down in a chair, nonambulatory, to a patient who is up walking around and happy, but this is unfortunately a transient experience in most. As far as our ability to produce normal children following surgery, radiation therapy, and chemotherapy is concerned, I think that it would be no different than we presently are doing with present modes of treatment. I think the long-term sequelae of chemotherapy in the children that we have dealt with have been minimal. I think the children that have been cured with Wilm's tumor and with rhabdomyosarcomas, which in our institution has gone from 10% to 90% cures for localized tumor, have tolerated the chemotherapy well.

Discussant.   You talk about the role of chemotherapeutic agents in simply treating residual disease, what about the role of chemotherapeutic agents as radiosensitizing agents?

Dr. Newton.   I think there are a number of approaches, and this is one. We know that the addition of actinomycin D to radiation therapy does things. I think it might be possible to improve radiation therapy, for example, by the interaction of actinomycin D on the brain tumor cell along with the radiotherapy. It might be that we can achieve greater effects from the radiation therapy by having an additional effect from a radiosensitizer such as actinomycin D. And I think these are the considerations which I think will have to be made and perhaps will be factors which could be added to other effective chemotherapeutic agents. I think that one of the lessons that have been learned in chemotherapy is that we don't deal usually now with one drug. Usually, it's a multiple drug approach. And I think also multidrug therapy regimens will need to be implemented, one of which might be actinomycin D to act along with the radiotherapy.

Dr. Seydel.   Are there are comments on the part of the speakers regarding this?

Dr. Kramer.   I just want to make one point clear. One of the things I was trying to say was that I think it would be very wrong at this point when you really don't know what is very good or what damage we are causing to indiscriminately add chemotherapy to the modes of treatment already established. I think this has to be done in a prospective controlled clinical trial. I think it is essential that these things be worked out under controlled conditions where we can judge the effect. We can determine that these patients are better, how many are better for how long, and what is the potential damage we are storing up. I think to simply go into a clinical situation when we don't have any good evidence would be wrong. When I say prospective I don't necessarily mean treating people prospectively for subclinical disease. I mean a controlled clinical trial where we can truly evaluate the effects.

Dr. Katz.   I think there was some evidence at one time that BCNU given along with x-ray therapy might be beneficial. Would you comment on that?

Dr. Newton.   I refer to Dr. Walker's experience in which he showed definitely this was the case and that the average survival went from about 20 weeks to 40 weeks, I believe. Is that what you referred to? We are using CCNU or methyl-CCNU because it is easier to give. It is apparently about as effective.

Dr. Katz.   In the first round of therapy though?

Dr. Newton.   We are presently considering a multidrug regimen in which we have just started a series in a fashion that Dr. Kramer outlined.

Treatment of Pituitary Tumors by Radiation Therapy

Simon Kramer, M.D.,

Professor and Chairman,
Department of Radiation Therapy
and Nuclear Medicine,
Thomas Jefferson University Hospital,
Philadelphia, Pennsylvania

The treatment of pituitary tumors is a subject of particular interest to radiation therapists. These tumors are the only remaining large group of benign tumors that radiation therapists commonly treat, and since patients with these tumors have a tendency to stay alive for long periods of time, they are ideally suited to the measurement of any possible damage that radiation therapy must cause.

CHROMOPHOBE ADENOMAS

Chromophobe adenomas are, of course, the most common of the pituitary tumors. They are often considered to be non-hormone-producing, but many patients have been seen with histologically proven chromophobe adenomas that do produce hormones. Of particular interest in this regard is a relatively small group of patients with amenorrhea and galactorrhea and very high prolactin levels, who are included in the series of patients discussed here but who will also be considered as a separate group.

Today it is well established that radiation therapy plays a major role in the management of chromophobe adenomas. The question is not whether to use radiation therapy but rather how best to use it—in conjunction with surgery or as the sole method of treatment? In an attempt to answer this question, I should like to consider the patients with chromophobe adenoma that we have seen at Thomas Jefferson University Hospital over the last 16 years or so.

Symptoms

The symptomatology for chromophobe adenomas is well known. Impairment of the visual fields and visual acuity is among the most striking features, then the occurrence of headaches and symptoms of hypopituitarism and hypothalamic impairment such as somnolence, obesity, impotence, and amenorrhea. The age incidence is primarily in the second, third, and fourth decades, but there can be a very wide range; in our series the youngest patient was 11 years and the oldest 87 years.

Treatment Techniques

These patients have all been treated by the same technique, which is used at Jefferson for all pituitary and parapituitary tumors. This technique involves an arc rotation situated in the coronal plane. By changing the arc angle, the volume of high-dose irradiation may be changed appropriately. Figure 1 shows an isodose distribution taken with a 180° arc. There is fairly even irradiation encompassing the target volume. It is a very simple technique that can be made even more elegant by rotating a 180° arc with a wedge, which can be changed in direction at the 90° level, thereby developing a volume that is totally homogenous as far as dose is concerned.

When, occasionally, for some reason, rotation cannot be employed, we use a three-field technique (Fig. 2), which is essentially the same as the arc technique. By use of wedges in the lateral fields the dose can be evenly distributed; without wedges the high-volume dose extends above the pituitary region. It can be seen that the tumor dose is considerably higher than the dose given to most of the normal brain.

A third technique is mentioned merely to condemn it. The use of parallel opposed fields for treatment of pituitary tumors is poor because considerable volumes of tem-

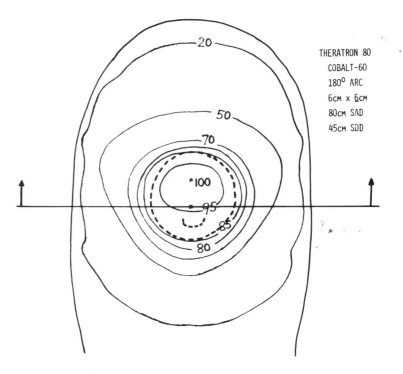

Fig. 1. A typical isodose distribution for a 180° rotational field.

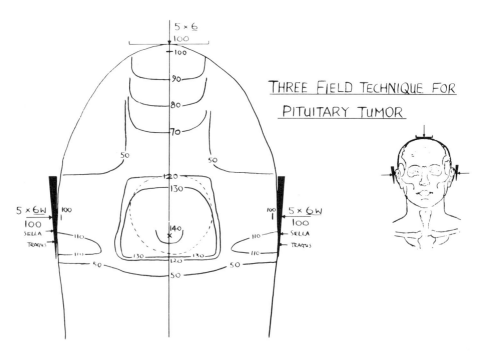

Fig. 2. Three-field technique using two lateral wedges and a superior open field. (Reprinted, with permission, from reference 1.)

94

poral lobe receive a somewhat higher dose (an appreciably higher dose in some areas) than the target volume itself.

Our treatment of pituitary tumors calls for daily fractionation of 200 rads per day, 5 days a week, to a total dose of 4500–4600 rads. We had used this dose initially for all pituitary tumors, but have advanced our dose for the acromegalies to 5000 rads in 5 weeks in an attempt to bring about a more rapid reduction of the growth hormone level; however, 4500–4600 rads is very satisfactory for the chromophobe adenomas.

Patients Treated on Clinical Diagnosis

Our series, from 1956 until about October, 1972, numbers 143 patients. About one-third have been treated on the basis of a clinical diagnosis only, without surgery; about two-thirds were treated postoperatively, and a small number were originally sent to us for a recurrent tumor (Table 1).

Wherever possible, it is worthwhile and necessary in most patients to establish a histologic diagnosis. This can best be done by a transsphenoidal approach. At the same time any cyst found can be emptied. Such a cyst is present in some 30% of patients with chromophobe adenomas. After the diagnosis has been established in this manner, radiation therapy may be initiated.

For a variety of reasons, a group of our patients (Table 2) have been treated on clinical grounds. These cases were treated for the most part in the days before the transsphenoidal approach was available. Also included in this group are some patients who had no visual difficulties, but whose disturbances were entirely endocrinological. These patients account for the great discrepancy between the male and female population in the group treated on the basis of clinical diagnosis, since they are mostly women with amenorrhea and galactorrhea. There were 12 such patients with galactorrhea and amenorrhea—young women, who were usually referred by the endocrinologist because of sterility problems. In those patients we have felt that treatment by radiation therapy without a biopsy was justified.

Of the whole group of 37 patients, about two-thirds, or a little less, are alive and well, giving an absolute survival rate of about 62% (Table 3). In this particular group the determinate figures are relevant because many died of other causes and some are lost to followup. The overall determinate survival figure for this whole group, from 1 to 16 years, is 82%. Of those that were treated more than 5 years ago (Table 3), about two-thirds are alive in the determinate group.

TABLE 1. TOTAL EXPERIENCE: CHROMOPHOBE
ADENOMA OF THE PITUITARY,
THOMAS JEFFERSON UNIVERSITY
HOSPITAL, 1956–1972

Basis for Treatment	Male	Female	Total
Treated on clinical diagnosis	10	27	37
Treated postoperatively	40	51	91
Treated for recurrence	10	5	15
Total	60	83	143

TABLE 2. CHROMOPHOBE ADENOMA OF THE PITUITARY TREATED BY
RADIATION THERAPY ON THE BASIS OF CLINICAL DIAGNOSIS

Number of cases	37
Advanced in age (67–81 years)	8
Patients with galactorrhea and amenorrhea	12
Present status	
Alive, no evidence of disease	
(1–16 year after treatment)	22
Alive, with post-surgical defect	1
Dead of other causes	8
Recurrence	4 (3 at 1 year; 1 at 6 months)
1 dead of other cause at 8 years;	
1 alive with no evidence of disease at 3 years;	
1 alive with defect at 1 year;	
1 died at operation	
Dead of disease	1
Lost to followup	1 (at 1 year, 2 months)

Patients Treated Postoperatively

The largest group in our series are those treated by postoperative radiation. These patients were treated by craniotomy (67) or a transsphenoidal approach (24) and of these, at least 30 were cystic (Table 4). Of the total number of 91, about two-thirds are alive without evidence of disease, and 9 patients, about 10%, are alive with deficit, a deficit usually caused by the craniotomy approach. These are patients who have developed third-nerve paresis, blindness in one eye, or hemiparesis, but are alive and apparently free of their tumor. A rather large number of patients have been lost to followup. Of the whole group, the absolute survival rate (1–16 years) is 75%, and the determinate survival rate 90% (Table 4).

Essentially there is no great change in the recurrence rate with time. In the group of 74 patients treated more than 3 years ago (Table 5), there were no recurrences what-

TABLE 3. CHROMOPHOBE ADENOMAS OF THE PITUITARY TREATED BY
RADIATION THERAPY ON THE BASIS OF CLINICAL DIAGNOSIS

	Treated	
Present Status	> 5 years ago	> 10 years ago
Alive, no evidence of disease	12 (2 later lost to followup)	6 (1 lost to followup after 10 years)
Dead of other causes	8	7 (4 aged 67–72 years)
Recurrence	2	2 (at 1 year)[a]
Dead of disease	1	1 (aged 74 years; at 4 years)

[a] One died at operation; the other died of other cause at 8 years.

TABLE 4. CHROMOPHOBE ADENOMA OF
THE PITUITARY TREATED BY
RADIATION THERAPY
POSTOPERATIVELY

Number of Cases	91
Postcraniotomy	67
Transsphenoidal biopsy	24
Found to be cystic—30	
Present Status	
Alive, no evidence of disease	60
Alive, with deficit	9
Lost to followup (< 1 yr)	8
Dead of other causes	7
Dead of disease	6
Recurrence	1
Absolute survival	69/91 or 75.8%
Determinate survival	69/76 or 90.8%

soever, an absolute survival rate of 73%, and a determinate survival rate of 90%. As to those treated more than 5 years ago, there are still no recurrences in a group of 57 patients. In the 27 patients treated more than 10 years ago, of course, the absolute survival rate is much lower. Many of these patients are old and have died of unrelated causes; 5 have been lost to followup after 5 years, and 2 rather more rapidly; some have died, after long intervals, of other causes. But 3 patients died with the disease at 5

TABLE 5. CHROMOPHOBE ADENOMAS OF THE PITUITARY TREATED BY
RADIATION THERAPY POSTOPERATIVELY

	Treated		
	> 3 years ago	> 5 years ago	> 10 years ago
Total cases	74	57	27
Present status			
Alive, no evidence of disease	47	33	10
Alive, with deficit	7	5	3
Lost to followup	8	9	7
	(<1 year)	(3 at <1 year; 6 at 3–4½ years)	(2 at <1 year; 5 at 5–8 years)
Dead of other causes	6	4	4 (at 4, 7, 8, 10 years)
Recurrences	0	0	0
Absolute survival	54/74 or 73%	38/57 or 66.6%	13/27 or 48%
Determinate survival	54/60 or 90%	38/44 or 83.3%	13/16 or 81%

months, 1 year, and 2 years. The determinate survival rate for a group of patients treated more than 10 years ago was about 80%.

Patients Treated for Recurrence

Another group are those treated for recurrence. Fifteen patients were referred to us from our own or other institutions after a recurrence was diagnosed (Table 6). In 11 patients the initial treatment was surgical without postoperative irradiation. Of those that had no postoperative irradiation, 8 recurred within 5 years and 3 were late recurrences. Two patients received some postoperative irradiation; they recurred at 8 years and at 17 years. Two patients had tumors which had been treated initially by radiation therapy alone, one of which recurred rather promptly and the other, in spite of a low-dose irradiation, which recurred after 17 years.

The results in these patients, treated for recurrence (Table 7), are not, of course, nearly as good. This group has an absolute survival rate of 40% and a determinate survival rate of 46%. Clearly, results with this group are by far the worst.

Patients with Galactorrhea

A subgroup of patients treated for chromophobe adenoma are those with galactorrhea (Table 8). These are primarily young women who have menstrual irregularities or amenorrhea; they describe galactorrhea as often present for many years, and they usually come to us for investigation of sterility. They usually do not have a very large pituitary fossa, although there is almost invariably evidence of some enlargement of the

TABLE 6. RECURRENT CHROMO-
PHOBE ADENOMA OF
THE PITUITARY,
THOMAS JEFFERSON
UNIVERSITY HOSPITAL,
1956–1972

Total number of recurrences	15
Male	10
Female	5
Treated initially by craniotomy	13
No postoperative radiation therapy	11
Recurred < 2 years	5
Recurred 3–5 years	3
Recurred > 5 years	3
Postoperative radiation therapy	2
Recurred at 8 years	1
Recurred at 17 years	1
Treated initially by radiation only	2
Recurred at 2 years	1
Recurred at 17 years	1
(Treatment: 2800 rads)	

TABLE 7.   OUTCOME: RECURRENT CHROMOPHOBE ADENOMA

Total number of recurrences	15
Treated initially by craniotomy	13
Alive, no evidence of disease	2 (10 years; 2½ years)
Alive, no evidence of disease but later lost to followup	2 (5 years; 2½ years)
Dead of other cause	1 (6½ years)
Alive with deficit	1 (11 years)
Recurrence	1 (5 years)
(Retreated and alive with no evidence of disease at 8 years)	
Lost to followup (< 1 year)	2
No improvement, dead of disease	3 (8 years; 4 years; 1 year)
Died during radiation therapy	1
Treated initially by radiation only	2
No improvement, dead of disease	1 (1 year)
Alive, no evidence of disease	1

sella. Twelve of these patients were treated on the basis of clinical diagnosis, and all of these were treated before assays of prolactin levels were available. Eleven of these patients have done well. There has been no progression in the enlargement of the sella. In all but one of them galactorrhea has disappeared, but none of them has returned to normal menstruation. One of these patients has conceived after having been given cycling drugs, and many other of these patients are on cycling drugs. In every other respect these patients are well, and they have had no further evidence of tumor growth, with the exception of one male patient. He had a very large pituitary tumor with an enormously high prolactin level, in excess of 2000 ng/ml. At operation he was found to have a large invasive tumor. He did well after radiation therapy for a very short period of time, but rapidly recurred with chiasmal syndrome. Upon reoperation, he was found to have a

TABLE 8.   OUTCOME:CHROMOPHOBE ADENOMA OF THE PITUITARY

Patients with galactorrhea	17
Treated on clinical diagnosis	12
Alive, no evidence of disease	11
Dead, with second brain tumor (at 1 year, 6 months)	1
Treated postoperatively	4
Alive, no evidence of disease (3 years–6 years, 4 months)	3
Recurrence (at 5 months)	1
Treated for recurrence	1
Alive, no evidence of disease (at 2 years, 6 months)	

huge recurrence. He is now alive a year after his second operation and doing well. One patient, in whom there was visual disturbance with marked impairment of visual fields and acuity, had had two craniotomies. Upon a third recurrence of her visual difficulties, she was referred to us; she is now alive and well 2½ years later without evidence of galactorrhea or visual defects.

Complications

We have reviewed our patients carefully to try to discover any ill effects of radiation therapy in this group, but have failed to discover any morbidity of either visual pathways or cerebral function. Nor have we observed any impairment of pituitary function attributable to irradiation. However, just recently we have seen a patient treated solely by radiation therapy for a chromophobe adenoma, who developed pituitary hypofunction 9 months after her treatment. As this has happened in only one of 143 patients, it is clearly a very rare complication.

We have found it difficult to make a quantitative assessment of the degree of improvement in visual acuity or visual fields as the result of radiation therapy, especially in patients treated postoperatively; in these cases it is impossible to apportion the benefit derived from surgery and that derived from postoperative therapy. A number of patients show immediate improvement after their operation, but in others the improvement occurs after a variable period of time. The overall results, however, show that 80% of our patients treated either postoperatively or by radiation alone can return to full work capacity and lead useful lives.

Discussion

Conventional radiation therapy in the doses indicated is safe and satisfactory. The need for radiation therapy is established by the fact that patients treated by surgery alone have a high recurrence rate. Both control rates and functional results are worse in patients treated for such recurrences than in patients given irradiation initially.

Having concluded that radiation therapy is indeed necessary for these patients, the second question to be settled is whether these patients should be treated by radiation therapy alone or whether they should receive postoperative radiation. The removal of a chromophobe adenoma by craniotomy has an appreciable operative morbidity. Some 10% of our operated patients have significant postoperative deficits. This can be avoided by treating the patients primarily by radiation therapy.

On the other hand, surgery does provide histopathological proof of the tumor and thus prevents the misdiagnosis of a craniopharyngioma as a chromophobe adenoma (less than 15% of craniopharyngiomas show neurological evidence of calcification). Although these tumors respond well to radiation therapy, we have shown that a much higher dose is needed for cure.[1] One-third of our tumors treated surgically were found to be cystic. There is evidence that cystic tumors treated initially by radiation therapy do less well more often; this may be because these cysts are under pressure and the cells surrounding them may well be hypoxic and therefore less responsive to irradiation. Surgical emptying of the cyst will relieve the pressure and therefore the hypoxia. Finally our series of patients treated primarily by radiation therapy have shown a low but definite recurrence rate (4 of 37 patients). However, only 1 of 91 patients is known to have recurred when treated by combined surgery and radiation therapy. Should a recurrence take place after adequate irradiation (4500 rads in 4¼ weeks) further radiation therapy would entail a high risk of brain necrosis and would therefore be contraindicated. Thus, reliance must then be placed on surgical removal of the recurrence.

Nevertheless, there are certain clinical situations when treatment by radiation therapy without prior biopsy is indicated.

Firstly, in elderly patients and patients in poor general condition, when the transsphenoidal approach is not available. The low risk of a recurrence is more than outweighed by the risk of craniotomy, provided always that vision is not acutely threatened. If vision is so threatened, a surgical decompression is mandatory.

Secondly, the group of young women mentioned previously with prolactin-secreting tumors. These patients usually have small tumors and no visual symptoms. They do well with radiation therapy alone.

Finally, there is a group of patients with extremely large chromophobe tumors and long-standing visual defects. In these patients craniotomy carries a high risk both for morbidity and mortality. Since visual deterioration has been present in these patients for a long time, decompression is unlikely to improve them. Operative mortality has been estimated as high as 30–40%, and the risk of further deterioration following surgery may reach 60%. In this situation, treatment aims at preserving residual vision and even here occasionally remarkable improvement can occur. Three patients in this category have been seen by us recently. The first patient with a history of visual impairment over several years was found to have a massive tumor, with almost complete destruction of the pituitary fossa, displacement of the carotid arteries, and elevation of the anterior cerebral arteries. The basilar artery was displaced posteriorly (Figs. 3a–3c). In view of the considerations mentioned above, treatment by radiation therapy alone was selected. The patient's visual defect did not improve, but 2 months after completion of therapy residual vision remained stable. Because of the lack of improvement, craniotomy was performed and the patient died postoperatively. The second patient also had a tremendous tumor (Figs. 4a and 4b). This patient, a surgeon, had abandoned his work for over 1½ years prior to seeking advice. He was still able to read with the help of a magnifying glass. Again, treatment by radiation alone was selected. His visual defect remained unchanged. Dissatisfied with this result, he underwent craniotomy 2 months after completion of therapy and became totally blind and decerebrate postoperatively. A third patient also had a massive lesion with total destruction of the clivus and the pituitary fossa (Figs. 5a–5c). This patient had a 5-year history of progressive visual loss and was almost blind when seen by us. She, too, was submitted to radiation therapy without prior decompression. This patient regained useful vision and can now continue to care for herself 1½ years after her treatment. It must be emphasized once more that in these desperate situations treatment is designed primarily to prevent further visual deterioration without undue risk of morbidity or mortality.

Conventional radiation therapy is firmly established in the treatment of chromophobe adenomas of the pituitary gland. A dose of 4500 rads to the target volume in 4½ weeks given in 22 fractions appears to give excellent results in terms of local control with a minimum occurrence of morbidity. It goes without saying that full neurological and endocrinological studies must be completed before the method of treatment is selected. The neurological investigation must include an air-contrast study so that the size of the tumor can be determined and the possibility of empty sella syndrome excluded. This syndrome can produce all the symptoms of a sellar tumor, but obviously requires

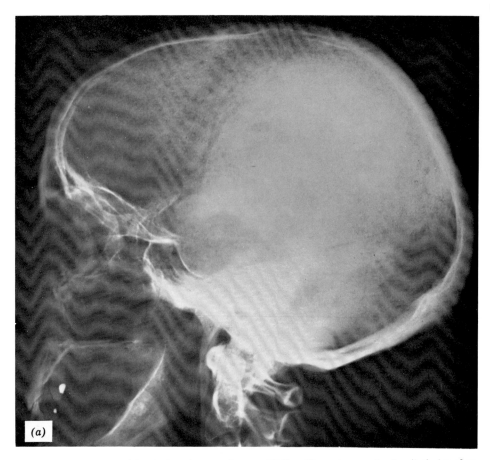

(a)

Fig. 3. (*a*) Destruction of the pituitary fossa can be seen. (*b*) Carotid arteriogram showing displacing of anterior cerebral artery. (*c*) Posterior displacement of the basilar artery can be seen.

different management. Carotid and, when indicated, vertebral arteriography should be done as well. In most patients it is desirable to have histologic confirmation of the tumor and, if a large cyst is present, it should be emptied prior to irradiation of the tumor. This can be done best by the transsphenoidal approach which eliminates much of the risk of morbidity inherent in craniotomy in these patients. Only when vision is acutely threatened should this risk be accepted. And with specific groups, namely, patients who are old or in poor general condition, patients with predominantly endocrine symptomatology without visual disturbances, and patients with very large tumors and long-standing visual impairment, radiation therapy alone may well be the best form of therapy available.

ACROMEGALY

Radiation therapy has long been used in repeated low doses (about 1000 rads) to suppress the common symptoms of acromegaly, such as acroid changes and changes in visual field and acuity. Over the past 25 years a single course of irradiation to a higher

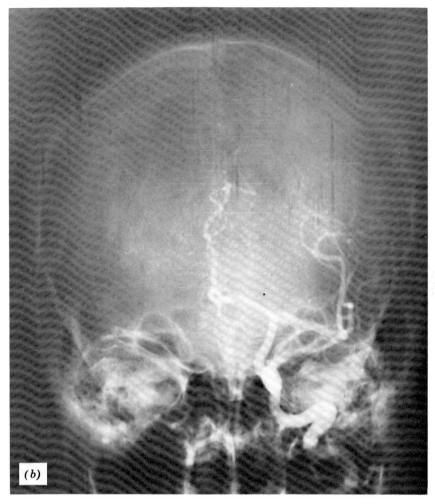

(b)

Fig. 3.   (Continued)

dose has become accepted as a means of permanently halting the disease, with less undesirable side effects than the formerly used treatment. Our usual practice in treating
eosinophil adenomas is to deliver 5000 rads in 5 weeks in daily 200-rad fractions 5
times per week, a dose that has proved to be entirely safe and that may bring about a
faster and more consistent decrease in the human growth hormone (HGH) levels than
lower doses.

HGH levels are invariably elevated in acromegalic patients. Previously it has been
claimed that conventional radiation therapy does not reduce the HGH levels to normal,
although it may arrest tumor growth.[2] Our results,[1] however, as well as those reported
by others[3, 4] have shown serum HGH levels, as measured by radioimmunoassay, to
return to normal or near-normal levels after conventional irradiation with 4500–5000
rads. This decrease does, however, take several months and sometimes as long as 1–2
years to become evident. Because serious side effects are rarely seen with irradiation
and because it is effective in arresting the disease, we feel it is the preferred treatment

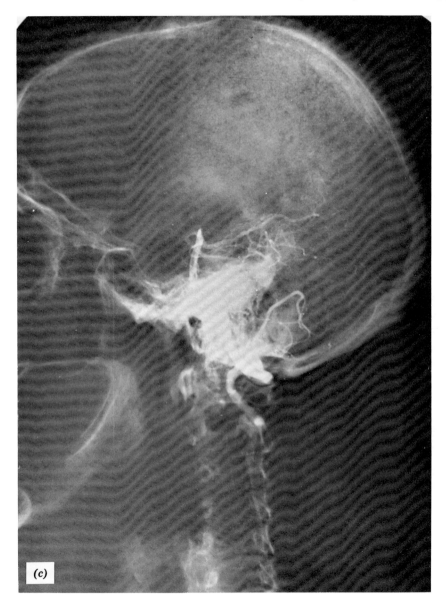

Fig. 3.   (Continued)

for acromegaly. In cases in which the HGH level is extremely high and a delay of 6 months to 2 years for reduction is unacceptable, a surgical procedure, which reportedly will bring about a faster HGH level decrease, may be needed. Likewise, preirradiation surgery is called for in patients suffering severe curtailment of visual acuity or showing evidence of hemorrhage in the pituitary tumor.

At Thomas Jefferson University Hospital we have treated 29 patients for acromegaly over the past 16 years, all but one of whom were treated on the basis of the clinical

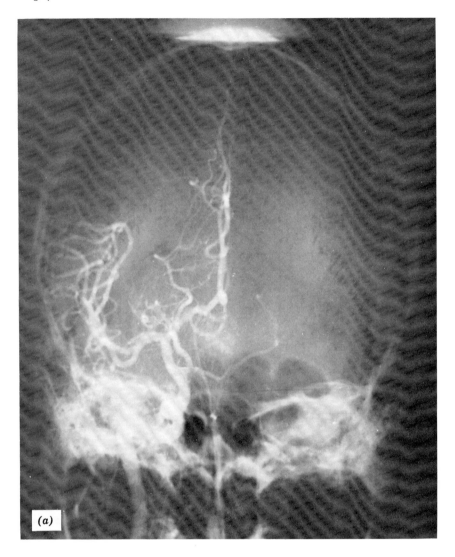

Fig. 4.   Pneumoencephalogram showing (*a*) superior displacement of anterior cerebral artery; (*b*) tumor filling lower portion of third ventricle.

diagnosis. This patient was treated after a craniotomy for a presumed chromophobe adenoma, which then histologically proved to be an eosinophil adenoma. Two patients received 4000 rads or less; the other 27 received approximately 4500–5000 rads (Table 9). Twenty-five of the total group of 29 have shown no clinical evidence of recurrence, giving a failure rate of 14% (4/29). Of the 4 patients who have died in the group of 25 recurrence-free cases (Table 10), 1 died of suspected hypopituitarism 5 years after treatment. She was a patient who refused further care after irradiation. Another of these 4 suffered a coronary occlusion at 3 years, 5 months, after treatment; 1 died of myocardial infarction at 2 years, and 1 ruptured his splenic artery at 1 year.

Three of the 4 patients who showed evidence of recurrence (Table 11) were treated

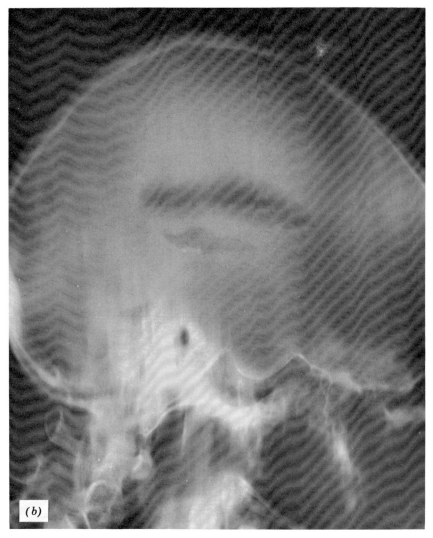

Fig. 4.   (Continued)

subsequently by craniotomy and hypophysectomy and the fourth was treated by stereotaxic transsphenoidal hypophysectomy. There were no postoperative complications in any of these cases. Two are alive and show no evidence of disease, one at 5 years postoperatively and 8 years post radiation therapy, the other at 11 years postoperatively and 11 years, 4 months, post radiation therapy; the third died of unknown cause at 1 year, 3 months, postoperatively and 6 years post radiation therapy, and the fourth was lost to followup at 2 years postoperatively and 5 years post radiation therapy.

HGH studies were made for all but 9 of these 20 patients, these having been treated before serum HGH radioimmunoassays had become available.

Pre- and posttherapy studies were made in 8 patients (Table 12). Pretherapy the fasting levels in these patients ranged from 13 to 37 ng/ml and maximum levels, as

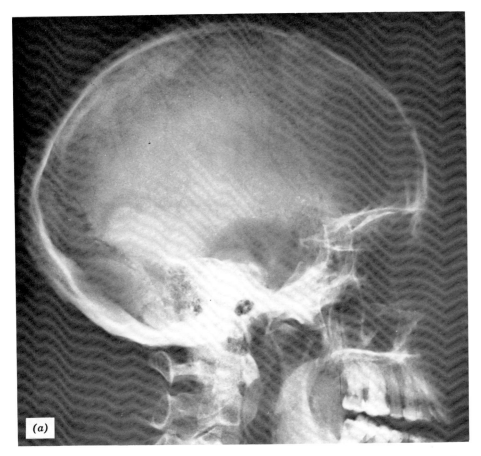

Fig. 5. (a) Destruction of pituitary fossa can be seen. (Reprinted, with permission, from reference 1.) (b) Submento-vertical view of skull showing destruction of clivus. (Reprinted, with permission, from reference 1.) (c) Pneumoencephalogram showing extent of tumor in third ventricle. (Reprinted, with permission, from reference 1.)

measured at the time of a glucose tolerance curve, were between 22 and 73 ng/ml. Within 9 months to 2 years posttherapy, the HGH levels had returned to normal in 7 of the 8 patients, with fasting levels of 4–10 ng/ml and maximum levels of 8–9.9 ng/ml. (In our laboratory, the normal levels are considered to be: for the male, resting, 0–2.5 ng/ml, and after mild exercise, 0–4.5 ng/ml; for the female, resting, 0.5–20.5 ng/ml and after mild exercise, 3.5–20.0 ng/ml.) One of the 8 patients still has an elevated HGH level 1 year, 1 month after therapy, but even in this patient there has been a marked decrease from the posttherapy level. Details of these cases are given in Table 12a.

Posttherapy studies only were performed in 8 patients, in all of whom HGH levels (both fasting and maximum) have returned to normal (Table 13). In 1 patient HGH levels were studied only pretherapy; this patient, who had evidence of acromegaly for 27 years before therapy, died of myocardial infarct 2 years after treatment without any further HGH test being made. Details of these 9 patients are given in Table 13a.

HGH levels were studied in 3 of the 4 patients with clinical evidence of recurrence

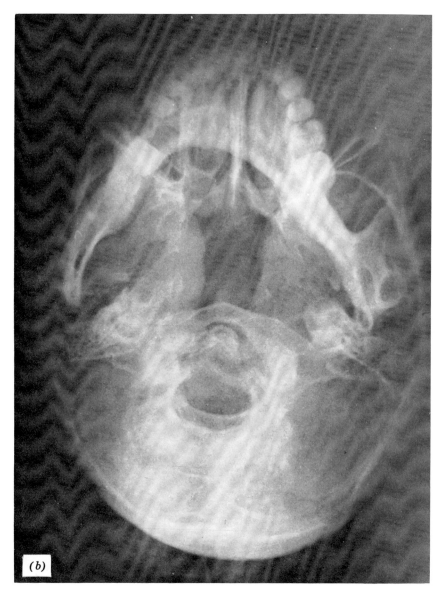

Fig. 5. (Continued)

(Table 14). In 1 patient, posthypophysectomy levels only were studied and were found to be normal at 6 and 10 years postoperatively. Levels in the other 2 patients were studied at the time of recurrence and posthypophysectomy. The levels for these 2 patients were still elevated at 3 and 5 months, respectively, postoperation, but had returned to normal at 4 years for the patient for whom the data are available.

Sixteen out of the 20 patients studied for HGH levels have shown no evidence of recurrence, and in all but 1 of these 16, HGH levels have returned to normal; the remaining patient has shown a marked decrease in HGH level at 1 year, 1 month,

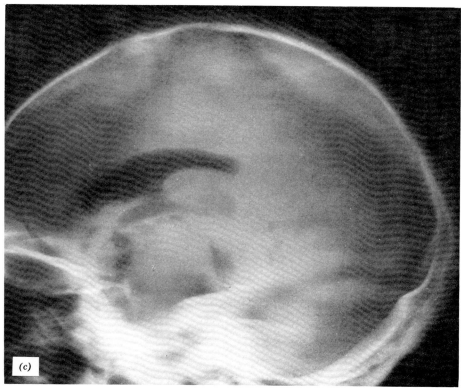

Fig. 5. (Continued)

TABLE 9. ACROMEGALY, THOMAS
JEFFERSON UNIVERSITY
HOSPITAL, 1957–1971[a]

Total number of patients	29
Treated on clinical diagnosis	28
Treated postcraniotomy	1

Treatment

Tumor doses (rads)	Number of patients
≤ 4000	2
4400–4600	20
≥ 5000	7

Factors: Co[60]   SA distance, 80 cm
160–220° arc rotation
Field size, 4.5 × 4.5 to 6.5 × 6.5 cm
1000 rads/week, five 200-rad fractions

Results

No clinical evidence of recurrence	25
Clinical evidence of recurrence	4
Failure rate	4/29 or 14%

[a] Reprinted, with permission, from reference 1.

TABLE 10. CASES OF ACROMEGALY WITH NO
CLINICAL EVIDENCE OF RECURRENCE[a]

Total number	25
Alive with no evidence of disease	21
>10 years	5/7
>5 years	12/16 or 75%
>3 years	17/21 or 81%
<3 years	4
Dead	4
1 hypopituitarism (?) at 5 years, 6 months	
1 coronary occlusion at 3 years, 5 months	
1 ruptured splenic artery at 1 year	
1 myocardial infarct at 2 years	

[a] Reprinted, with permission, from reference 1.

TABLE 11. CASES OF ACROMEGALY WITH
CLINICAL EVIDENCE OF
RECURRENCE[a]

Number of cases	4
Treated by craniotomy and hypophysectomy	3
Treated by stereotaxic hypophysectomy	1
Alive with no evidence of disease	
At 5 years postoperatively, 8 years postradiation	1
At 11 years postoperatively, 11 years, 4 months postradiation	1
Dead (cause unknown)	
At 1 year, 3 months postoperatively, 6 years postradiation	1
Lost to followup	
At 2 years postoperatively, 5 years postradiation	1

[a] Reprinted, with permission, from reference 1.

TABLE 12.   ACROMEGALY: HUMAN GROWTH HORMONE
STUDIES

A. Cases not studied (1957–1966)	9
B. Cases studied pre- and posttherapy	8
Pretherapy HGH Levels (ng/ml)	
Fasting	13–37
Maximum (glucose tolerance)	22–73
Post-therapy HGH Levels (ng/ml)	
Return to normal (9 months to 2 years)	7/8
Fasting	4–10
Maximum	8–9.9
Still elevated (1 year, 1 month)	1/8
Fasting	17.8
	(pretherapy: 37)
Maximum	20
	(pretherapy: 60)

[a] Reprinted, with permission, from reference 1.

TABLE 12a. DETAILS OF 8 CASES OF ACROMEGALY: GROWTH HORMONE LEVELS STUDIED PRE- AND POSTTHERAPY[a]

Patient	Present Status		HGH Levels (ng)					Replacement Therapy	Complications
	Condition	Years post-therapy	Pretherapy		Posttherapy				
			Fasting	Maximum	Years post-therapy	Fasting	Maximum		
D.G.	Alive and well	5	23	31.5	$1\frac{1}{2}$	13	19	Thyroid diabinase, cortisone	None
					$1\frac{3}{4}$	4	8		
C.W.	Alive and well	$3\frac{1}{2}$	37	60	2	17.8	20.0	None	None
B.L.	Alive with partial vision	3	45	73	1	25	25	Thyroid, cortisone	Very poor vision bilateral. Craniotomy—no tumor; optic nerve vasculitis
					$1\frac{3}{4}$	3.5			
M.C.	Alive and well	3	27	46	$\frac{2}{3}$	28		None; cortisone for asthma	None
					1	16			
					2	5			
M.C.	Alive and well	$2\frac{1}{2}$	24	31	$2\frac{1}{4}$	9.5		None	Central scotoma right eye
L.P.	Alive with memory loss	$2\frac{1}{3}$	13	40	1	9		None	Marked memory loss
					$1\frac{5}{6}$	4.2			
I.T.	Alive and well	$1\frac{1}{2}$		22	$1\frac{1}{2}$	5.5		None	None
V.D.	Alive and well	1	40	40	$\frac{3}{4}$	10	9.9	Oricon	None

[a] Reprinted, with permission, from reference 1.

TABLE 13. CASES OF ACROMEGALY: HUMAN GROWTH HORMONE STUDIES[a]

C. Cases studied posttherapy only (1959–1970)	8
Posttherapy HGH Levels (ng/ml)	
Normal levels (2 years, 7 months to 13 years)	8
Fasting	1.2–14
Maximum	4–12.5
D. Cases studied pretherapy only (1967)[b]	1
Pretherapy HGH levels (ng/ml)	
Fasting	33
Maximum	33.2

[a] Reprinted, with permission, from reference 1.
[b] Died 2 years later.

TABLE 13a. DETAILS OF 8 CASES OF ACROMEGALY: GROWTH HORMONE LEVELS STUDIED POSTTHERAPY ONLY[a]

Patients	Present Status		HGH Levels (ng)			Replacement Therapy
	Condi-tion	Years post-therapy	Years post-therapy	Fasting	Maximum	
D.B.	Alive and well	13⅓	11	9.5	12.5	None
Q.F.	Alive and well	12	12	4	7	None; empty sella syndrome
M.J.G.	Alive and well	9	9	3	4	Chlomophene
M.K.	Alive and well	8¾	6	3	4	None
			8	3.4		
E.F.	Alive and well	7	7	1.2		None
H.F.	Alive, no vision left eye, post-cranio-tomy	5	5	1.2		Cortisone, thryoid postcraniotomy
C.C.	Alive and well	3¾	3¾	6		None
I.B.	Alive and well	3	3	14		None (insulin)

[a] Reprinted, with permission, from reference 1.

TABLE 14. ACROMEGALY: HUMAN GROWTH HORMONE STUDIES

E. Patients with clinical evidence of recurrent acromegaly   3[b]
    Cases studied posthypophysectomy only   1

HGH Levels (ng)	6 years postoperatively	10 years postoperatively
Fasting	5	2
Maximum	9	

Cases studied at time of
recurrence and post-
hypophysectomy

	Patient E.S.			Patient J.S.	
HGH Levels	Prehypo physec- tomy	Three months post- operatively	Four years post- operatively	Prehypo- physec- tomy	Five months post- operatively
Fasting	92	32	10	49	27.5
Maximum	132	80	—	—	30.0

[a] Reprinted, with permission, from 1.
[b] Three out of four such patients were studied.

TABLE 15. CASES OF ACROMEGALY: ENDOCRINE
            REPLACEMENT THERAPY

Patients treated by radiation alone	22
No replacement therapy	17
Replacement therapy	5
1 thyroid	
2 chlomophene, oricon	
1 cortisone, thyroid, diabinase pre- and postradiation	
1 insulin	
Patients who underwent craniotomy/hypophysectomy	7
(1 diagnosis, 2 suspected recurrences, 4 recurrences)	
No replacement therapy (no tumor found at craniotomy)	1
Replacement therapy (all on cortisone and thyroid)	6

[a] Reprinted, with permission, from reference 1.

posttherapy. On the other hand, 2 of the 4 patients who showed evidence of recurrence had elevated HGH levels. Thus HGH levels seem to parallel the clinical condition of the patient.

Replacement therapy was needed for only 5 of the 22 patients treated by radiation therapy alone and only 1 of these 5 required cortisone. He was found to suffer from panhypopituitarism prior to treatment. Of the 7 patients who had a craniotomy, hypophysectomy, or both (1 for diagnostic purposes; 2 for suspected, but not subsequently confirmed, recurrences; 4 for what were found to be recurrences), only 1 patient (one of the two in whom no tumor was found) does not require replacement therapy; the other 6 receive cortisone and thyroid hormone (Table 15).

In 4 patients there has been morbidity, presumably caused by the irradiation. In one of these patients severe impairment of vision occurred 6 months after radiation therapy. No cause of this visual deficiency could be found, there was no recurrence of the tumor, and optic nerve vasculitis was diagnosed by exclusion. In another of these 4 patients a central scotoma in the right eye developed 9 months after therapy and has remained unchanged for 2 years. This patient also suffers recurrent headaches as the result of an empty sella syndrome, as does the third of these 4 patients. A marked memory loss has occurred in the last of these patients 1 year after therapy; this patient has no other neurological abnormality, but is unable to work.

As can be seen from the foregoing data, most of our patients with acromegaly responded well to conventional radiation therapy and continue well; HGH levels return to normal between 6 months and 2 years after treatment, few patients require replacement therapy, and morbidity from such treatment is rare. Thus, radiation therapy would seem to be the treatment of choice in acromegaly, as well as in patients with chromophobe adenomas.

REFERENCES

1. Kramer, S. Indications for, and Results of, Treatment of Pituitary Tumors by External Radiation. In Kohler, P. O., and Ross, J. T., Eds., *Diagnosis and Treatment of Pituitary Tumors, Excerpta Medica, Amsterdam, 1973, p. 217.*

2. Roth, J., S. M. Glick, P. Cuatrecasas, et al: Acromegaly and Other Disorders of Growth Hormone Secretion. *Ann. Intal. Med.* **66**:760–768 (1967).

3. Lawrence, A. M., S. M. Pinsky, and I. D. Goldfine: Conventional Radiation Therapy in Acromegaly: A Review and Reassessment. *Arch. Internal. Med.* **128**:369–377 (1971).

4. Roth, J., P. Gordon, and K. Brace: The Efficacy of Conventional Pituitary Irradiation in Acromegaly. *New Engl. J. Med.* **282**:1385–1391 (1970).

Radiation Therapy of Acromegaly and Nonsecretory Chromophobe Adenomas of the Pituitary

Glenn E. Sheline, Ph.D., M.D.,
Professor of Radiology
Division of Radiation Oncology,
University of California,
San Francisco Medical Center,
San Francosco, California

William M. Wara, M.D.,
Assistant Professor of
Radiation Oncology,
University of California,
San Francisco Medical Center,
San Francisco California

CONVENTIONAL RADIATION THERAPY IN THE TREATMENT OF ACROMEGALY

Although more than six decades have passed since the first reported use of irradiation in treatment of acromegaly,[1, 2] the indications for this form of therapy remain in doubt. It is well established that modern conventional radiation therapy is associated with minimal morbidity, including lack of suppression of normal pituitary function, but we do not know how to predict which patients will respond satisfactorily, how long a time must lapse before response becomes evident, nor how important a rapid response is.

Before an assay for growth hormone was available, radiation therapy was widely accepted as the treatment of choice for acromegaly. The results, as judged by the effects of growth hormone on target organs and tissues and by pressure effects of the pituitary tumor, were generally considered good. There was, however, frequent failure to reverse soft-tissue changes. When a reliable growth hormone assay became available, it was soon noted that, after treatment by irradiation, the fasting growth hormone (FGH) level does not rapidly return to the normal range. Whether this evidence should have assumed the paramount importance it has may be debated; nevertheless, in many medical centers, conventional irradiation for treatment of acromegaly was virtually discarded. Other treatment methods such as transsphenoidal cryohypophysectomy (TCH) and high-dose, heavy-particle, irradiation replaced conventional irradiation. These new methods, however, cannot be applied to all patients, are not always successful, and may even result in a significant morbidity, including reduction of function in the anterior pituitary.

In 1970, Roth, Gordon, and Brace[3] reported that in 20 patients at 1–2 years after treatment with conventional radiation therapy, the mean fall of plasma growth hormone concentration was 51% and that in 7 patients studied between $2\frac{1}{2}$ and 4 years, the mean drop was 76%. Nevertheless, even with the large percentage decreases, 4 of the 7 studied at the later time still had abnormally high FGH levels. These investigators were unable to relate response to initial FGH level, volume of sella, or duration of disease. They concluded that although the efficacy of conventional irradiation was the same as that for all other modalities of therapy, the side effects were fewer. Lawrence, Pinsky, and Goldfine,[4] in 1971, presented data on the FGH levels of 16 patients irradiated before 1965 and 12 irradiated thereafter. In 13 (81%) of the 16 earlier patients, the acromegaly was judged clinically inactive and the FGH levels were 10 ng/ml or less. Of the 12 patients who had both preirradiation and postirradiation FGH determinations, 9 had values in the normal range 6 months to 4 years after treatment. The 3 failures in this group were among the 6 patients with preirradiation FGH levels above 40 ng/ml. Lawrence, Pinsky, and Goldfine concluded that external radiation therapy continues to be appropriate therapy for this disease. Recently Kramer[5] reported on the successful treatment with conventional external radiation therapy of 7 of 8 patients. Success was substantiated by preirradiation and postirradiation FGH determinations.

We too have been interested in reevaluating the role of conventional radiation therapy. In this context, conventional radiation therapy is that given by external photon irradiation. Although the radiation source and dose–time pattern may vary and are included in this definition, radiation sources implanted into the lesion and the use of particle irradiation are excluded. We shall first present a brief review of results in patients given conventional radiation therapy before use of the growth hormone assay.

These results include posttreatment growth hormone levels for 17 of the 24 of our patients who are still living and for 28 patients treated elsewhere. We shall then present results of a survey of several institutions in which patients have received primary radiation therapy and have had pretreatment growth hormone evaluation. Finally, a small group of recently irradiated patients who previously failed to respond satisfactorily to transsphenoidal cryohypophysectomy will be considered.

Review of Patients Treated Before the FGH Assay

From 1942 to 1959, 37 patients with laboratory and clinical evidence of active acromegaly were treated with conventional radiation therapy at the University of California, San Francisco (UCSF).[6] Of this group 41% had sufficient extrasellar extension of the tumor to produce a visual field defect. Results presented in 1961 were judged on the basis of endocrine activity and pressure effects. Evaluation of endocrine activity was based on metabolic rate, carbohydrate tolerance, serum phosphorus level, adrenal activity (as measured by 17-ketosteriod and 17-hydroxysteroid excretion), and growth of skeletal and soft tissues. Reversal of chemical abnormalities and arrest of soft-tissue changes were accepted as a successful result. Pressure effects, judged separately, were considered controlled if there was improvement in visual fields, cessation of headaches, and no additional expansion of the sella.

The results of conventional radiation therapy for acromegaly in these patients treated before 1960 are shown in Table 1. Both endocrine hyperactivity and pressure effects were controlled in about three-fourths of the patients treated with radiation doses greater than 3500 rads. Patients receiving lower doses, unless retreated, experienced a markedly lower control rate, namely, about 25%. Ten of the 15 patients with abnormal pretreatment visual fields had normal posttreatment fields. There were no complications and no evidence of increased hypopituitarism in patients treated with a single course of irradiation, even though doses in some patients were as high as 6000 rads. No patient thought to be controlled has shown evidence of reactivation of the disease.

Of our patients treated with conventional radiation therapy prior to 1965, 24 (more than half) are alive. Seven of these, all of whom are reportedly clinically asymptomatic, are at remote distances and could not be reevaluated. The other 17 have been restudied and FGH levels obtained. These data are shown in Fig. 1a. At the time of restudy 13 of the 17 patients were clinically without evidence of active acromegaly and had normal

TABLE 1. CONVENTIONAL RADIATION THERAPY FOR
ACROMEGALY

	Fraction Patients Controlled	
Controlled by	Dose $\leq$ 3500 rads	Dose $>$ 3500 rads
Initial treatment		
Endocrine hyperactivity	5/19 (26%)	13/17 (77%)
Pressure effects	5/17 (29%)	14/18 (78%)
Retreatment	7/19	none
Total controlled	12/19 (63%)	14/18 (78%)

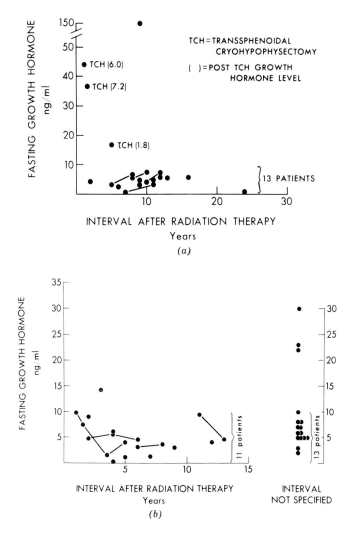

Fig. 1.   Fasting growth hormone levels of patients treated by conventional radiation therapy. Multiple determinations for a single patient are connected by lines. (a) Patients treated at our institution; (b) patients treated elsewhere.

FGH levels (≤ 7.5 ng/ml). In 10 patients the FGH concentration was <5 ng/ml. Of the 4 patients with elevated FGH levels, 2 underwent transsphenoidal cryohypophysectomy (TCH) 12–14 months after radiation therapy. The FGH levels after TCH were reduced to normal (data in parentheses in Fig. 1a) in both patients; in retrospect, however, it is evident that their surgical treatment was too soon after radiotherapy to evaluate the effectiveness of the irradiation. Of the 2 cases that were clear-cut radiation failures, 1 was salvaged by means of surgical intervention, performed 5 years postirradiation; the other patient has acromegaly that is uncontrolled clinically and chemically and he refuses additional treatment.

Figure 1b shows the postirradiation FGH concentrations, as a function of time after treatment, for 12 patients treated at other institutions (who will be discussed below).

Eleven of the 12 patients were considered to have normal posttherapy FGH values. The data reported by Lawrence, Pinsky, and Goldfine are shown, for comparison, on the right side of the figure. Combining the data of Fig. 1a and 1b (including that of Lawrence and co-workers) reveals that 37 of 45 (82%) patients developed normal FGH concentrations and that 2 of the 8 considered to be failures may have undergone surgical treatment too soon for evaluation. These data provide little information about the rapidity of decrease of the FGH level.

Patients Treated After Advent of FGH Assay

We have had few previously untreated acromegalic patients referred to us for primary radiation therapy since 1965 when the FGH assay became available at UCSF. Therefore, in order to gain more patient material for analysis, we conducted a survey of radiotherapists at each of 49 institutions throughout the country that comprise the Radiation Therapy Oncology Group (RTOG). Thirty-four responded, but only 8* had data useful for our purpose. For the data to be considered useful the minimal requirements were: (1) the patient was treated only with conventional radiation therapy, with a dose of at least 4000 rads; (2) pretreatment and posttreatment FGH levels were available; and (3) possible complications, including treatment-induced hypopituitarism, could be evaluated. Most of the patients had data relating to diabetes mellitus, diabetes insipidus, adrenal function, thyroid function, and visual fields.

Figure 2 shows the preirradiation and postirradiation FGH concentrations for 18 patients obtained through the RTOG survey and for the 12 previously reported by Lawrence and co-workers. The RTOG data are shown as solid circles and solid lines, whereas the Lawrence data are given as open circles and broken lines. Patients with pretherapy levels of ≤45 ng/ml are depicted in Fig. 2a and those with higher levels in Fig. 2b. The FGH levels usually decreased with time posttherapy, and most levels eventually reached the normal range. Because observations were infrequent, it is not possible in many patients to determine when the FGH concentration reached normal. Although the number of patients with measurements at later times is limited, none of those in whom the FGH level dropped below 10 ng/ml have subsequently risen above that level.

The data, including that of Lawrence, Pinsky, and Goldfine, from Fig. 2 are analyzed in Table 2. Implicit in this table is the assumption that once the FGH concentration drops below 10 ng/ml it remains below 10. The results for those patients with pretherapy levels of 45 ng/ml or less are as follows: At 12 months posttherapy, 7 of 19 patients had achieved FGH levels of less than 10, and by 24 months 14 of 17 had achieved such an FGH level (it should be noted that the 3 who failed to achieve an FGH level of less than 10 have a follow-up period of less than 3 years). Ten patients had initial FGH concentrations of 50 ng/ml or greater. Of these 10, 5 FGH values dropped to 10 or less within 1 year. However, 2 patients, observed as long as 3 years, had persistently elevated values, namely, 25 and 65 ng/ml.

Although the above observations relate only to FGH concentrations, considerable other data were obtained from the RTOG survey. However, the data supplied differed

* Contributors, in addition to the present authors, were Drs. H. C. Berry (University of Washington), M. S. Lee (Rush Presbyterian–St. Luke's Medical Center), M. J. Wizenberg (University of Maryland), W. N. Brand (Northwestern Memorial Hospital), M. Griem (University of Chicago), S. Kramer (Jefferson Medical School), and D. Pistenma (Stanford University).

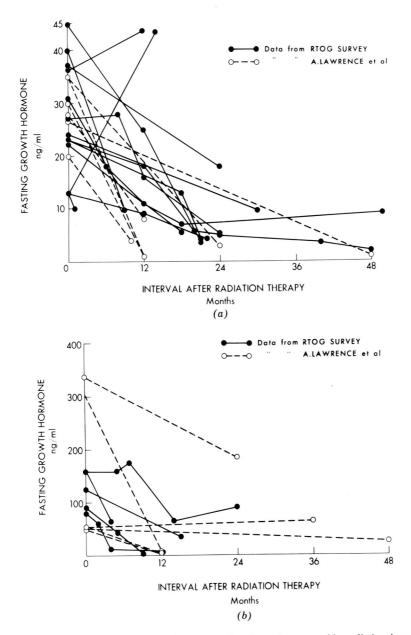

Fig. 2. Pretreatment and posttreatment FGH concentrations for patients treated by radiation therapy alone. Multiple determinations for a single patient are connected by lines. (a) Patients with initial concentrations of 45 ng/ml or less; (b) patients with initial concentrations of 50 ng/ml or more.

TABLE 2. FGH CONCENTRATION BEFORE AND AFTER
RADIATION THERAPY (RT)

FGH Level before RT (ng/ml)	Period after RT (months)	Patients in Whom FGH Decreased to ≤ 10 ng/ml
≤45	12	3/13 (4/6)[a]
	18	6/11 (4/6)
	24	9/11 (5/6)
	36	10/10 (6/6)
≤50	12	2/4 (3/6)
	18	2/3 (3/6)
	24	2/3 (3/6)
	36	2/2 (3/5)

[a] Data of Lawrence, Pinsky, and Goldfine are in parentheses.

from institution to institution in such a way that we were unable to assemble useful pretherapy and posttherapy information for such aspects as response of FGH levels to insulin and glucose administrations, glucose tolerance, and other clinical and laboratory parameters indicative of acromegalic activity.

Radiation Therapy of TCH Failures

Approximately 25% of patients with acromegaly treated by transsphenoidal cryohypophysectomy at UCSF have failed to achieve normal FGH levels. The failures have been predominately in those with pretreatment FGH values above 40 ng/ml. During the last year, 9 such patients have been referred for conventional external radiation therapy and have received pituitary doses of 5000 rads, given in 5 fractions per week with 180 rads per fraction using a 4-MeV linear accelerator and treating two fields per day. In 2 of the 4 patients for whom we have follow-up data (Table 3), the FGH concentration decreased by 50% within 2 and 7 months after radiation therapy.

TABLE 3. RADIATION THERAPY (RT) FOR TRANSSPHENOIDAL
CRYOHYPOPHYSECTOMY FAILURES

Patient	FGH Level before TCH (ng/ml)	Period TCH to RT (months)	FGH Levels	
			Before RT (ng/ml)	After RT (ng/ml)
O.D.	80	5	35	17 (2 months) 14 (12 months)
L.S.	54	24	20	15 (8 months)
J.S.	35	12	25	12 (7 months)
J.W.	70	12	20	23 (8 months)

TABLE 4. CRANIOTOMY AND RADIATION
THERAPY

	FGH Concentration (ng/ml)	
Patient	Pretherapy	Posttherapy
C. Q.	57	36 (9 months)
		8 (19 months)
E. B.	106	21 (27 months)
B. Q.	200	72 (15 months)
S. S.	54	34 (4 months)
		14 (16 months)
		6 (31 months)
A. B.	130	1.2 (12 months)

Without solicitation, 1 of these patients (O. D.) described improvement, including decrease in shoe and ring size, before completion of her radiation therapy. FGH levels of the other 2 patients have not changed significantly 8 months after irradiation. We conclude that some TCH failures may be salvaged by conventional radiation therapy.

Combined Craniotomy and Radiation Therapy

Recently, 5 patients with acromegaly and large suprasellar extension of the pituitary tumor have been treated by craniotomy with partial resection of the adenoma followed by radiation therapy. The early results may be of interest (Table 4). Three of these now have normal FGH concentrations and the other 2 have shown reductions of 64 and 80%.

Remarks

To conclude, conventional radiation therapy probably is as effective in the primary control of acromegaly as any other form of therapy. Second, with properly administered radiation therapy, there is minimal morbidity and no cases of secondary hypoadrenalism have been documented. Third, the length of time required for control has not been well studied but appears to vary from a few months to at least 2 years. Although there are no data available indicating the necessity for more rapid control, it seems reasonable to think that the more rapid the better, but only if the faster method carries no significant increase in mortality or morbidity. Fourth, conventional radiotherapy may also be an effective means of treating the acromegalic patient who has failed to respond to surgical methods or who is known to carry a high risk of failure. Lastly, we believe well-designed studies are now necessary to evaluate more fully the proper place of conventional radiation therapy, the indications for planned combined surgical and irradiative procedures, and the use of irradiation following surgical failure.

NONSECRETORY CHROMOPHOBE ADENOMAS

Between 1933 and 1968, 140 patients received primary treatment for chromophobe adenoma at the University of California, San Francisco (Table 5).[7] During this period, 3 treatment regimens were used: 23 patients were treated with radiation therapy alone (RT), 37 by surgical decompression with biopsy and partial removal of the adenoma (S), and 80 by partial surgical resection plus postoperative radiation therapy (S+RT).

In general, radiation, whether given as primary therapy or postoperative, was delivered by means of bilateral, opposed fields using energy photon beams of 1 MeV or more, with radiation doses to the pituitary of 4000–5000 rads. Overall treatment time was usually 5–6 weeks, with 5 fractions per week. Exceptions to this treatment policy occurred during the early period, when 14 patients were treated with lower energy x-rays, and 18 received doses of 1700–4000 rads. Except for 2 patients, in whom the surgical procedure was carried out by means of the transsphenoidal approach, all surgical patients underwent craniotomy.

Four of the 23 patients treated by radiation therapy alone had histologic confirmation of the diagnosis. In 1 patient, biopsy material was obtained from the nasopharyngeal extension of the adenoma; in the other 3 it was obtained at craniotomy (2 performed because of radiation failure and 1 because of a small bulge of the tentorium seen on a repeat pneumoencephalogram that was done because of a carotid aneurysm). All 19 patients without a histologic diagnosis had enlarged, eroded sellae, 15 had hypopituitarism, and none had the type of calcification characteristic of a craniopharyngioma. Visual field defects, consistent with a suprasellar mass, were present in 15 of these 19 patients. Each of the 4 patients with normal visual fields had pneumoencephalographic evidence of a suprasellar mass. As will be seen later, 67% of those patients with visual field defects showed improvement following irradiation, indicating that their lesions were radiosensitive and thus not aneurysms. It seems reasonable to assume that the presumptive diagnosis of chromophobe adenoma was correct in nearly all, if not all, of the 19 patients who did not undergo biopsy.

Table 6 indicates the reasons for use of radiation therapy without preceding biopsy or decompression. Patients considered as poor surgical risks were generally of advanced age; 35% of the RT patients were over 60 years of age as compared with 12% of those

TABLE 5. INITIAL FINDINGS

Abnormality	Number of Patients			
	RT (23 patients)	S (37 patients)	S + RT (80 patients)	Total (140 patients)
Visual field defect	18 (78%)	36 (97%)	75 (93%)	129
Enlarged sella	23 (100%)	35 (95%)	77 (96%)	135
Hypopituitarism	16	17[a]	41[a]	74
Into nasopharynx	1	0	1	2
Local invasion	—	7	5	12

[a] Underreported, as many patients underwent surgical management before pituitary function was completely assessed.

TABLE 6.   REASON FOR TREATMENT
WITH RADIATION ONLY

Reason	Number of Patients
Surgery refused	5
Poor risk	7
Normal visual fields	5[a]
Minimal field deficit	2
Unknown	4
Total	23

[a] One biopsied later; other 4 had small suprasellar extensions.

undergoing surgical procedures. Visual fields were normal in 22% of the RT patients
compared with 5% for those treated surgically. Thus there was a tendency to use radiation therapy as the only treatment for patients of advanced age, for those considered
poor surgical risks, and for a selected group with minimal or no visual field deficit.

Results and Discussion

An adenoma was considered to be controlled as long as further growth was not evident
and any improvement achieved by the treatment was maintained. Primary reliance was
placed on serial determinations of visual fields, performed by a neuroophthalmologist.
We have not seen, in the absence of visual field changes, recurrence manifested by
decreasing pituitary function or increasing sellar expansion. We have seen 2 instances
of increased visual field defects associated with an "empty sella," without recurrence of
the adenoma. In the analysis of results each eye was considered separately.

Excluding eyes with normal pretreatment visual fields, treatment resulted in some
degree of improvement in 68% of patients treated by RT and in 58% of those in whom
surgical decompression was used. This difference is probably explained by the fact that
the surgical patients tended to have more extensive visual defects.

Table 7 represents an attempt to circumvent the bias introduced by the tendency to
utilize surgical decompression when the deficits were large. In this table, consideration

TABLE 7.   RESPONSE FOR EYES WITH DEFICIT $\leq \frac{1}{2}$ VISUAL FIELD

Visual Field after Therapy	Treatment Group Response (%)			
	RT	S	S + RT	S and S + RT
Normal	36	43	41	41
Improved	32	43	16	22
No change	32	3	33	27
Worse	0	11	10	10

is limited to patients with eyes having relatively early and approximately comparable deficits, that is, deficit present but involving one-half or less of the visual field. Normal fields followed therapy in 36% of those patients treated by radiation alone and in 41% of those treated by surgical decompression. Improvement, but without return to normal fields, followed treatment in 32% of the RT group and 22% of the group having surgical decompression. Thus, improvement of pretreatment defects, involving one-half or less of the visual field, occurred in 68% of the RT group and 63% of the combined S and S+RT groups. The only apparent difference in the early response to treatment for these groups is that 10% of the surgery patients had a permanent increase in the defect.

The present status of all treated patients is summarized in Table 8. Of the 23 RT patients, 12 are under observation and without evidence of recurrence. Eight* patients without evidence of recurrence have died of intercurrent disease, and 1 refuses to return for study. The high rate of death from intercurrent disease was because many of the elderly patients selected for RT had other, nonrelated, medical problems at the time. The 2 recurrences were in patients treated with relatively low radiation doses during the earlier part of the study period.

Patients treated by surgery alone (S) have shown a high recurrence rate. Of the 29 patients who survived the surgical procedure, 20 (69%) have had a definite recurrence, 1 has died of intercurrent disease, and 5 have been lost to followup. Only 3 of this group are known to have no recurrence.

Of the 80 patients treated by S + RT, 57 (71%) are living and their disease is under control, 14 have died of intercurrent disease without evidence of recurrence, and 9 (11%) had adenomas that have recurred. Time of recurrence has varied from a few months to 12 years.

Absolute and determinate control rates for the various treatment groups are presented in Table 9. The *absolute rate* includes all patients. The *determinate rate* excludes patients who died as a result of the surgical procedure as well as those dead of intercurrent disease or lost to followup. Disregarding patients who died of intercurrent disease biases the results in favor of RT, but removal of patients dying postoperatively or lost to followup provides a bias in favor of surgery. As will be seen, the conclusions to be reached are the same whether the absolute or the determinate rate is used.

TABLE 8. CURRENT STATUS

| | Number of Patients | | |
Status	RT	S	S + RT
No recurrence			
Under observation	12	3	57
Dead from intercurrent disease	8	1	14
Lost to follow-up study	1	5	0
Recurrence	2[a]	20	9
Surgical death	—	8	—

[a] Treated with doses of 1720 and 1900 rads.

* Includes the 1 who underwent a surgical procedure because of a known carotid aneurysm.

TABLE 9.   CONTROL RATES

Interval (years)	Absolute Control Rate			Determinate Control Rate		
	RT	S	S + RT	RT	S	S + RT
2	18/21	18/37	77/80	18/18	18/26	77/79
5	14/15	9/36	65/72	14/15	9/24	65/68
10	5/7	3/32	37/47	5/5	3/21	37/43
15	2/3	0/25	20/31	2/2	0/16	20/27
20	1/3	0/23	11/17	1/1	0/14	11/15

For periods up to 10 years, there was no difference in the absolute control rates for those patients treated with RT as compared with those treated with S + RT. The determinate control rates are also similar for the 2 series in which radiation therapy was used. There are too few RT only patients observed longer than 10 years to permit comparison at later times.

Results for both the RT and S + RT groups are clearly better than those for the S only group at all intervals after treatment. For example, at 5 years the absolute control rates for the RT and the S + RT series are 93 and 90%, respectively, but only 25% for the S series. At 10 years, the absolute and determinate control rates for the S + RT series were, respectively, 79 and 86%, whereas, they were only 9 and 14% for the S group. By 15 years all patients treated only by surgery had had a recurrence, but two-thirds of those patients treated with S + RT were without recurrence, even at 20 years. Furthermore, it is probable that the late control rates in the irradiated patients would have been even higher if some of those treated during the early phase of the study period had received larger doses of irradiation.

With doses of 1720–3000 rads, 5 of 9 adenomas have recurred whereas only 5 patients of 85 treated with a dose of 4000 rads or more have shown evidence of recurrence (Table 10).

Complications.   After surgical decompression, the visual field deficit was permanently greater in 17 patients (Table 11). In each case the change was directly attributable to the surgical procedure. Seven patients, about 5% of those operated, experienced major damage to vision. In 4 patients with at least one-half of one or of both visual fields intact preoperatively, the end result was total blindness.

TABLE 10.   RECURRENCE VERSUS RADIATION DOSE

Dose (rads)	Number Treated		Known Recurrences	
	RT	S + RT	RT	S + RT
1720 to < 3000	2	7	2	3
3000 to < 4000	2	7	0	1
≥ 4000	19	66	0	5

TABLE 11. VISUAL FIELDS WORSE AFTER SURGICAL
TREATMENT

A. Minor change 12 eyes (10 patients)

B. Major change 10 eyes (7 patients)

Before Surgery	After Surgery
3 patients: bilateral hemianopsia	Bilateral blindness
1 patient: blind + hemianopsia	Bilateral blindness
3 patients: unilateral hemianopsia	Unilateral blindness

The major complications, other than damage to optic nerves, are shown in Table 12. There were 8 deaths due to the surgical procedure. This is 7% of all patients operated. In the 88 patients who underwent craniotomy since 1945, there have been 4 postoperative deaths:—one was due to a cerebral infarct and the other 3 involved adenomas that had extensive local invasion.

Cerebrospinal fluid (CSF) rhinorrhea occurred in 2 patients in whom the tumor had extended into the nasopharynx and in 1 in whom there was erosion through the floor of the sphenoid sinus. The 3 instances of severe brain damage were associated with lesions that extensively infiltrated brain, and it was not possible to determine whether the brain damage was due to the adenoma, the treatment, or both.

Other than epilation, usually transient, no complication has definitely been attributable to radiation therapy. One of the patients with CSF rhinorrhea was in the RT group, but his adenoma had extended into the nasopharynx, where it had been biopsied.

SUMMARY

One hundred and forty patients with chromophobe adenomas were treated by radiation therapy, surgical decompression, or surgical decompression followed by radiation

TABLE 12. OTHER COMPLICATIONS

Complication	Treatment Group		
	RT	S	S + RT
Operative deaths	—	8	—
Cerebrospinal fluid rhinorrhea	1[a]	0	2[b]
Wound infection	—	2	0
Severe brain damage	0	1[a]	2[a]
Cranial nerve injury	0	1[a]	1[a]

[a] Permanent.
[b] Transient.

therapy. The initial response of the visual fields was the same for each form of therapy. The control rates at all intervals from 2 to 20 years were, however, much greater when irradiation was given. At 10 years the absolute control rate was 71% for radiation therapy, 79% for decompression plus irradiation, but only 9% for surgery alone. After 10 years no patient without irradiation was free of recurrence.

Surgical procedures yielded a 7% mortality rate, and 5% of those operated who survived experienced major damage to optic nerves or chiasm. No major complication could be attributed to irradiation.

REFERENCES

1. Béclère, A. The Radio-therapeutic Treatment of Tumours of the Hypophysis, Gigantism, and Acromegaly. *Arch. Roentgen Ray, London* **14**:142–150, (1909-10).

2. Gramegna, A. Un cas d'acromégalie traité par la radiothérapie. Note clinique. *Rev. Neurol.* **17**:15–17 (1909).

3. Roth, J., Gorden, P., and Brace, K.: Efficacy of Conventional Pituitary Irradiation in Acromegaly. *New Engl. J. Med.* **282**:1385–1391 (June 18, 1970).

4. Lawrence, A. M., Pinsky, S. M., and Goldfine, I. D.: Conventional Radiation Therapy in Acromegaly. A Review and Reassessment. *Arch. Internal Med.* **128**:369–377 (September 1971).

5. Kramer, S.: Indications for, and Results of, Treatment of Pituitary Tumors by External Radiation. *In,* Diagnosis and Treatment of Pituitary Tumors, edited by P. O. Kohler and G. T. Ross. Amsterdam, Excerpta Medica, 1973. Pp. 217–230.

6. Sheline, G. E., Goldberg, M. B., and Feldman, R.: Pituitary Irradiation for Acromegaly. *Radiology* **76**:70–75 (January 1961).

7. Sheline, G. E.: The Treatment of Nonfunctioning Chromophobe Adenomas of the Pituitary. *Amer. J. Roentgenol. Radium Therapy Nucl. Med.* **120**:553–561, 1974.

Cryosurgery in the Treatment of Acromegaly

Seymour R. Levin, M.D.,
Chief, Metaboliic Unit, Wadsworth
Veterans Administration Hospital,
Los Angeles, California;
Assistant Professor of Medicine,
University of California,
Los Angeles, California

Though several methods are available for treating acromegaly, no method is uniformly effective in all patients. Furthermore, though growth hormone (GH) measurements are widely available and most procedures used will reduce GH, reliable indices of optimal overall endocrine and metabolic responses to any form of therapy have not been established. Studies of long-term effects of therapy on morbidity and mortality are in progress. However, criteria for the choice of initial treatment have, in general, not been developed.

One form of treatment, which has been used for the past decade, is stereotaxic, transsphenoidal cryohypophysectomy.[1-3] This procedure has been used at the University of California in San Francisco since 1965. Over 100 patients have been treated with this method at the San Francisco center. Data will be presented from the first 50 patients. In addition to the results of therapy, three other aspects will be discussed: (1) utilization of changes in carbohydrate metabolism as an index of response; (2) evaluation of preoperative factors that might give clues as to the eventual results of treatment; and (3) use of this information to help make an initial choice of treatment.

METHODS

The patients evaluated (25 men, 25 women, mean age 42 years) were admitted to the General Clinical Research Center. All patients had clinical criteria for acromegaly.[4] In addition, fasting serum growth hormone was elevated, usually above 10 ng/ml, and did not fall to less than 5 ng/ml 1 hour after 100 g oral glucose. General medical, endocrine, and radiological evaluation was performed[3] and, in the absence of suprasellar extension, patients were scheduled for cyrosurgery.

The details of the procedure have been previously reported.[2] The cryoprobe was inserted under guidance of the image intensifier as seen in Fig. 1.

Complications

These have been previously reviewed.[3] Table 1 demonstrates that most of the postoperative problems are transient, lasting a few days to a few weeks. Two patients with diplococcal meningitis occurring on the eighth and ninth postoperative day were treated successfully with penicillin. This complication has not occurred in the most recent 50 patients. Both patients with diabetes insipidus had remissions after several months.

RESULTS

Clinical Symptoms

Table 2 demonstrates the preoperative symptoms in the 50 patients. These symptoms appear to have developed over a period of years, as summarized in the table. Most prevalent were fatigue or lethargy, perspiration, and acral enlargement. Table 3 shows that, after surgery, some symptoms remitted, regardless of GH alteration. Other symptoms appeared related to lowering of GH to less than 10 ng/ml.

135

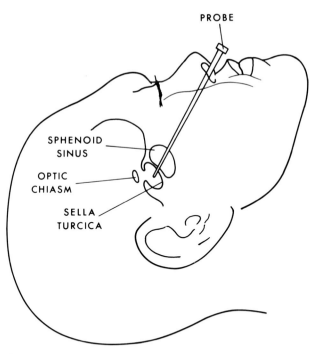

PROBE

SPHENOID
SINUS

OPTIC
CHIASM

SELLA
TURCICA

Fig. 1. Diagram of transsphenoidal approach to the pituitary gland with the cryohypophysectomy probe.

TABLE 1. COMPLICATIONS OF CRYOHYPOPHYSECTOMY

	Incidence/Total Patients
First 10 postoperative days	
Diabetes insipidus	10/50[a]
Hyponatremia	5/26[a]
Optic problems	9/50[ab]
CSF rhinorrhea	3/50[a]
Meningitis	2/50 (D. pneumonia)
Deaths	None
Late postoperative period (over 6 weeks)	
Adrenal insufficiency	6/50
Hypothyroidism	5/50
Diabetes insipidus	2/50

[a] Transient.

[b] 7 patients with paralysis of extraocular muscles, 2 patients with visual field defects (courtesy *California Medicine*[3]).

136

TABLE 2. SYMPTOMS IN ACROMEGALY FOR 50
PATIENTS

Symptom	Patients having symptom (%)
Earliest	
Fatigue or lethargy	82[a]
Paresthesias	62
Amenorrhea	32 (of females)
Headache	64
Later	
Excessive perspiration	88
Weight gain	76
Photophobia	46
Acral enlargement	96
Voice change	50
Decreased libido	27
Late	
Joint pain	76
Cardiac symptoms	12

[a] Indicates percentage of present 50 patient series having
particular symptom (courtesy *California Medicine*[3]).

TABLE 3. RELATIONSHIP OF ALTERATION OF
SYMPTOMS TO POSTOPERATIVE
GROWTH HORMONE LEVEL[a]

	< 10 ng/ml	> 10 ng/ml
Acral changes	53	33
Excessive perspiration	72	58
Decreased libido	33	0
Amenorrhea	29	0
Photophobia	31	0
Fatigue	33	33
Headaches	50	55
Arthralgias	56	55

[a] Values indicate percentage of patients with particular symptoms
that improved following cryohypophysectomy (courtesy, *California Medicine*[3]).

Growth Hormone Changes

Most recent postoperative follow-up examination was 6 weeks in 8 patients, 1 year in 17, 2 years in 11, 3 years in 11, and 4 years in 3. Preoperatively, mean GH was 52 $\pm$ 11 ng/ml (S.E.), and 10% had GH 10 ng/ml or less. At the most recent postoperative followup, mean GH was 17 $\pm$ 5 ng/ml ($p \leq .001$) and 76% of patients had GH 10 ng/ml or less.

Carbohydrate Balance

Table 4 demonstrates the changes in carbohydrate balance and relates these to altered GH.[5] Percentage of patients in the category that most closely approached normal, "GH less than 10 ng/ml and normal glucose tolerance," was increased 10-fold after surgery.

In 24 patients who had insulin levels measured (Fig. 2), postoperative insulin was less than preoperative during the 2-hour 100 gm oral glucose tolerance test given at the most recent follow-up exam (1 year or more). This also reflected improved carbohydrate metabolism as an index of response to lowered GH. Such changes were detectable as early as 6 weeks postoperatively.[5]

PROGNOSTIC INDICES

Lowering of GH

The group with postoperative GH 10 ng/ml or less (group A) was compared with the group having GH above 10 ng/ml (group B). Four major factors had a 20% greater prevalence in group B than in group A. These preoperative factors were: lateral sella area greater than 1.6 cm^2, fasting GH 50 ng/ml or more, fasting glucose > 90 mg/100 ml, and moderate to severe glucose intolerance.[5]

In 31 patients lateral sella outlines were drawn over pre- and postoperative skull films and areas were determined with a planimeter (Fig. 3). There was a significant

TABLE 4.   ALTERED CARBOHYDRATE METABOLISM
RELATED TO GH AFTER CRYOSURGERY
FOR ACROMEGALY FOR 50 PATIENTS[5]

	Fraction of Patients (%)	
	Preoperative	Postoperative[a]
Fasting GH > 10 ng/ml		
Normal glucose tolerance	38[b]	4
Glucose intolerant	52	19
Fasting GH < 10 ng/ml		
Normal glucose tolerance	6	60
Glucose intolerant	4	17

[a] At most recent follow-up examination (see text).
[b] Indicates percentage of 50 patients.

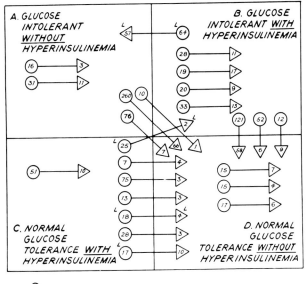

Fig. 2.   Evolution of glucose, insulin, and growth hormone after cryosurgery in 24 patients followed at least 1 year after treatment. Trend was for movement into the more normal category (*D*).

fall in this group in the lateral sella area postoperatively (films taken at least 1 year after surgery). Preoperative mean area was 1.6367 ± 0.1316 cm^2 (S.E.) and postoperative was 1.2967 ± 0.1005 cm^2 ($p < .001$). There was no mean difference between groups A and B, pre- or postoperatively. However, 63% of group B had preoperative lateral sella area more than 1.6 cm^2, whereas only 23% of those in group A had lateral sella areas above this size.[5]

In all but 4 out of 34 patients with preoperative GH less than 50 ng/ml, postoperative (most recent followup) GH fell to 10 ng/ml. On the other hand, only half of 16 patients with preoperative GH more than 50 ng/ml had postoperative GH 10 ng/ml or less.[5]

Patients with moderate or severe glucose intolerance had less impressive falls in GH. Ninety six percent of the group B patients had preoperative glucose intolerance, whereas only 42% of group A patients had preoperative glucose intolerance.[5] GH elevation rather than diabetic family history appeared most related to the glucose intolerance.[5]

DISCUSSION

Cryohypophysectomy is a form of therapy for acromegaly that rapidly lowers GH, with complications that are usually transient and manageable.

Factors that appear to favor a good endocrine–metabolic response to cryosurgery are moderate rather than large sella size, moderately rather than greatly elevated GH, and absence of severely disordered carbohydrate metabolism. Patients with such features

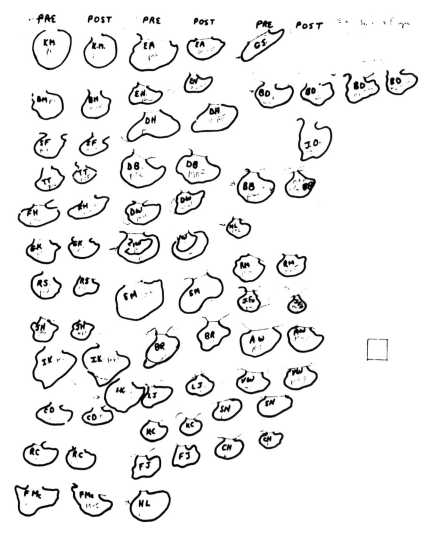

Fig. 3. Lateral sella drawings. Sella tracings in acromegalic patients before and at least 1 year after cryosurgery.

would be considered candidates for an optimal response to therapy, with falls in GH to 10 ng/ml or less, often accompanied by normalization of glucose tolerance.

We are presently exploring the possibility that preoperative patients with very large sellas, very high GH, and moderate to severe carbohydrate intolerance might received a more intense cryohypophysectomy (i.e., more than the usual 3 or 4 lesions). Also, such patients might get combinations of therapy as initial treatment. Presently, with Dr. Glenn Sheline, we are following a group of patients who have had cryosurgery without lowering of GH to 10 ng/ml or less. Dr. Sheline is using linear accelerator therapy.

We believe it is important in evaluating any response to therapy, to carefully assess hormonal, metabolic, and radiologic indices. Furthermore, with present radiological, surgical, and newer medical modalities,[6-8] it would seem desirable to retrospectively examine which features in patients seem to promote success or failure of each method.

Such investigations may help physicians choose initial therapy that will subsequently prove most adequate for reversal of abnormal metabolism and promotion of longevity.

SUMMARY

In 50 acromegalic patients cryohypophysectomy reduced GH so that 76% of those treated had postoperative GH of 10 ng/ml or less. Treatment was usually accompanied by more normal glucose tolerance and clinical improvement.

Preoperative patients with very large lateral sella area (over 1.6 cm²), very high GH (over 50 ng/ml), and severe glucose intolerance had less chance of optimal responses to cryosurgery than did those with moderately enlarged sellas, fasting GH under 50 ng/ml, and normal glucose tolerance or mild glucose intolerance.

Cryohypophysectomy works rapidly to relieve symptoms and lower GH. An approach has been presented that evaluates preoperative characteristics that can determine postoperative response. It is suggested that similar information be used in evaluating all forms of therapy, with the goal of improving the response to treatment.

ACKNOWLEDGMENTS

This work was performed when the author worked at the University of California, San Francisco, in association with Drs. Robert Seymour and John Adams of the Department of Neurosurgery, and Drs. Fred Hofeldt, Victor Schneider, Nathan Becker, Alan Rubin, Blake Tyrrell, and Peter Forsham of the Metabolic Research Unit, Department of Medicine, University of California, San Francisco.

REFERENCES

1. Rand, R. W.: Cryosurgery of the Pituitary in Acromegaly: Reduced Growth Hormone Levels Following Hypophysectomy in 13 Cases. *Ann. Surg.* **164**:587–592 (Oct. 1966).

2. Adams, J. E., Seymour, R. J., Earll, J. M., Tuck, M., Sparks, L. L., Forsham, P. H.: Transsphenoidal Cryohypophysectomy in Acromegaly: Clinical and Endocrinologic Evaluation. *J. Neurosurg.* **28**:100–104 (Jan. 1968).

3. Levin, S.: Manifestations and Treatment of Acromegaly. *Calif. Med.* **116**:57–64 (March 1972).

4. Davidoff, L. M.: Studies in Acromegaly. II. Historical Note. *Endocrinology* **10**:453–483 (1926).

5. Levin, S., Hofeldt, F., Schneider, V. Becker, N., Karam, J. H., Seymour, R., Adams, J., Forsham, P. H.: Cryohypophysectomy for Acromegaly: Factors Associated with Altered Endocrine Function and Carbohydrate Metabolism. Am. J. Med., Oct. 1974.

6. Lawrence, A. M., Kirsteins, L.: Progestins in the Medical Management of Active Acromegaly. *J. Clin. Endocrinol. Metab.* **30**:646–652 (May 1970).

7. Kolodny, H. D., Sherman, L., Singh, A., Kim, S., Benjamin, F.: Acromegaly Treated with chlorpromazine. *New Engl. J. Med.* **284**:819–822 (April 15, 1971).

8. Hall, R., Besser, G. M., Schally, A. V., Coy, D. H., Evered, D. Goldie, D. J., Kastin, A. J., McNeilly, A. S., Mortimer, C. H., Phenekos, C., Tunbridge, W. M. G., Weightman, D.: Action of Growth-Hormone-Release Inhibitory Hormone in Healthy Man and in Acromegaly. *Lancet* **2**:581–584 (Sept. 15, 1973).

A System of Therapy of Pituitary Tumors—Bragg Peak Proton Hypophysectomy

Raymond N. Kjellberg, M.D.,
Associate Clinical Professor of Surgery,
Harvard Medical School,
Cambridge, Massachusetts;
Visiting Neurosurgeon,
Massachusetts General Hospital,
Boston, Massachusetts

A system of therapy for pituitary tumors and other pituitary-related conditions has been developed and documented within the past decade to be virtually free of the risk of mortality and morbidity while achieving the therapeutic endocrinologic objective in about 9 out of 10 treated patients. The author reports experience with about 400 pituitary tumors and 250 other pituitary conditions (Fig. 1). Bragg peak proton therapy has no mortality and the earlier modest morbidity has been virtually eliminated. In particular we understand proton hypophysectomy to be the only means of restoring human growth hormone (HGH) or cortisol values to normal while preserving essentially normal pituitary function.

In the 400 pituitary tumors treated by all our methods, the sole procedure-related death occurred in 1962 in a transfrontally operated patient and was due to pulmonary embolus on the 12th postoperative day as the patient was prepared for discharge. Proton beam hypophysectomy is the method of choice. Transsphenoidal microsurgical hypophysectomy is favored over the transfrontal route. Radiofrequency hypophysectomy has been abandoned.

Our view of the problems of pituitary tumor therapy and our experience with the solutions will be presented.

PROBLEMS

Mortality

Cushing, the founding father of pituitary surgery and endocrinology, had in 338 patients an operative mortality of 5.5% and a patient mortality of 6.3%.[1] In his acromegalic patients, operation by the transsphenoidal route was associated with a mortality that was one-third that of the transfrontal route. The generation of neurosurgeons who followed Cushing devoted themselves largely to the transfrontal route. Ray reduced the operative mortality of transfrontal craniotomy in patients with chromophobe adenoma and acromegaly to 1.2% and 0%, respectively, or about 1% for both groups in his hands.[2, 3] However, operative mortality for the transfrontal route is more commonly 5–10%.

In our own experience, undesirable effects or complications of surgery with the potential for risk of death tend to be higher in transfrontally operated patients than in transsphenoidally operated patients (Fig. 2). Several of the complications are attributable to the use of general anesthesia. In fact, our only mortality directly attributable to the procedure, namely pulmonary embolus, is attributable to the anesthetized state rather than the cranial procedure *per se*.

Morbidity

Vision. Deterioration of visual acuity or fields is an outstanding risk associated with untreated pituitary tumors or with virtually all the methods by which pituitary tumors are treated. Progressive visual loss is often the specific reason for undertaking therapy, as is the case with chromophobe adenoma. On the other hand, the risk to vision during frontal craniotomy makes this a less desirable approach. In our experience, risk to

The project is supported by United States Public Health Service Grants CA 07368 and AM 04501.

vision by transsphenoidal microsurgical excision or proton hypophysectomy appears to have been reduced to very low levels.

During the first year (1963) of our clinical trial with the proton beam, we treated 3 cases of chromophobe adenoma with suprasellar extension of the tumor. We attempted radiation of the whole mass. Two of these patients had previously received substantial amounts of x-radiation. All 3 experienced significant visual loss 4–14 months following proton treatment. In addition, 1 died following craniotomy elsewhere, and we have been informed that the lesion was apparently malignant.[4]

Also in that year, we irradiated a girl with an unusual invasive pituitary lesion, considered to be a malignant connective tissue neoplasm. The beam diameter was large (51 mm), as was the dose (8000 rads). She lost all vision 15 months later, and at craniotomy, when no clear basis was found, we attributed the blindness to proton radiation. This risk was anticipated in what we regarded as a life-preserving effort.

These cases demonstrated problems associated with the application of proton radiation to cases that we came to realize were not suitable for the Bragg peak method.

1.   Patients with suprasellar extension of tumor are at risk. The paths of the optic nerves usually cannot be separated from the tumor by means of a pneumoencephalogram.

2.   Prior x-radiation contributes a hazard to proton therapy.

3.   Large-diameter beams in a single horizontal plane develop a wedge of overlap as they converge on the pituitary, such that the cumulative dose may be above tolerance for neural tissue.

Other than the above 4 early cases, none of the patients subsequently treated for

| | OPEN | | STEREOTACTIC | | |
	Frontal Craniotomy	Transsphen.	Transsphen. Radiofrequency	Bragg Peak Proton Beam	Total
Chromophobe Adenoma	10	6	1	44	61
Acromegaly	3	8	–	254	265
Cushing's Disease	3	2	–	56	61
Diabetic Retinopathy	16	–	7	183	206
Metas. Breast Carcinoma	1	1	4	30	36
Metas. Prostate Carcinoma	–	–	1	5	6
Suprasellar Meningioma	1	–	–	–	1
Misc. Pituitary Neoplasm	1	–	–	2	3
Other	–	3	–	–	3
TOTAL	*35*	*20*	*13*	*574*	*642*

7/1/73

Fig. 1.   Surgical procedures on the pituitary by Dr. R. N. Kjellberg.

| | OPEN | | STEREOTACTIC |
	Frontal Craniotomy	Transsphenoidal	Bragg Peak Proton Beam
NUMBERS OF PROCEDURES	19	12	323
WOUND INFECTION	0	0	0
CSF LEAK	0	1	0
COMA	0	0	0
SEIZURES –			
Major	0	0	0
Minor	0	0	4
DILANTIN INTOXICATION	1	0	0
PITUITARY INSUFFICIENCY			
Anterior Partial	0	0	7
Anterior Total	8	2	22
Posterior Permanent	0	0	0
Posterior Temporary	10	2	4
PULMONARY EMBOLISM	1 (died)	0	0
HEPATITIS	2	0	0
FURTHER TREATMENT	7	3	21

11/15/72

Fig. 2.   All pituitary procedures by Dr. R. N. Kjellberg—undesirable effects.

pituitary adenoma in our group has developed a visual handicap as the result of any of the therapeutic maneuvers employed. However, transfrontal craniotomy has produced many more partial alterations of visual function than transsphenoidal excision, where we have witnessed no decrease in visual acuity or fields in any instance. In 16 transfrontally operated patients, 4 experienced improvement in acuity and visual fields bilaterally. Three patients experienced improvement in visual function attributable to the improvement in one eye, but the other eye was worse. Both fields improved in 1 patient, but acuity remained the same; in 3 patients, both fields and acuity remained the same. Two patients have measurable decrements in either fields or acuity, but function at their preoperative levels of physical activity. We continue to regard risk to vision as an irreducible problem when the transfrontal route is employed.

By all forms of therapy—surgery, x-ray, and proton beam, patients are subject to visual loss due to the development of the so-called "empty sella syndrome."[5] This phenomenon appears to limit the ultimate success of intervention, but it also occurs without treatment, and it is fortunately rare.

Mental Status.   Alteration of mental status may be related to massive tumors, malignant invasions, or major endocrine disorders, and it represents another important risk of the transfrontal route of excision. We have not encountered complications of brain function related to transsphenoidal procedures. The only instance of temporary memory alteration was reported in our first proton-treated acromegalic patient and has not been observed again with the improved dosimetry of radiation.[6]

In our hospital, following a frontal craniotomy, a few patients have suffered delayed alteration of mental status. Patients have been noted to be bright and alert following transfrontal excision, then 2–5 days later, rather abruptly change and become poorly responsive. Angiography may reveal spasm of cerebral arteries. The hypothesis has been advanced that degenerating blood products in the subarachnoid space may be responsible.

Endocrine. Total surgical excision of a pituitary tumor inevitably obligates a patient to lifelong dependence on replacement medication. While this is normally satisfactorily managed as a modest inconvenience, the occasional inadvertent catastrophe in a stressed cortisone-dependent patient should be reckoned in the overall risk. Diabetes insipidus and its management are significant sources of disability to the patients. Deliberate subtotal excision may often avoid this inconvenience and risk. However, the patient frequently requires retreatment with x-ray or later reoperation to control persistent hyperfunction or recurrent mass. Microadenomas, tumors that are 10 mm or less in diameter, may be excised by the transsphenoidal microsurgical route, preserving the remainder of the gland. Such small tumors, however, represent a very small proportion of all adenomas, and the operative separation of larger tumors from normal pituitary cannot be reliably performed. Either total hypophysectomy or secondary therapy is normally required. Optimally, both hypopituitarism and high prospect of retreatment should and can be avoided.

Following conventional x-ray therapy, Glick found the values of HGH in acromegalic patients nearly identical before and after x-ray therapy.[7] We would not interpret his data as showing that x-ray had no effect. We think it is proper to credit the x-ray therapy with arresting the tendency for HGH levels to increase as they normally do. They did not, however, fall. The data of Roth et al on 20 cases requires greater care in interpretation.[8] In none of their 5 patients with postirradiation HGH values below 5 ng/ml (R. H., B. M., M. S., J. G., and J. J.) was any acral change observed. The value of one of these (J. G.) appears to have been 5 ng/ml before treatment, and the HGH values of 3 of the others appears to have been 6.5, 8, and 11 ng/ml. The degree of "activity" in these cases we would consider in doubt pending further information. Furthermore, in 2 of their 3 patients in whom acral regression was observed (G. S. and L. B.), the HGH levels were 39 and 28 ng/ml, respectively, after treatment. These very few patients (3 of 20, or 15%) demonstrating acral improvement have done so only between 2 and 4 years after treatment. However, as for the prospects for improvement beyond the second year after x-ray therapy, Glick's Fig. 2 shows 7 patients, 2 with no growth hormone decrease after 1 year (B. T. and W. S.), 3 with no 2-year measurement (G. S., A. T., and M. S.), 1 tested only at 12 and 30 months (M. M.), and only 1 (J. J.) with a decrease between 24 and 48 months. The "benefit" in that case is calculated by us to be another 10% of control or only 2 ng/ml.

There is a substantial body of evidence from Ray,[3] Adams,[9] Rand,[10] ourselves, and others that reduction of HGH below 5 or 10 ng/ml can be induced with substantially greater frequency, ranging from 50 to 75% of cases by the variety of means used by these authors. Furthermore, their experience and ours substantiates a strong correlation between levels of HGH in the normal range and remission of acral changes. We have observed acral regression when patients with "active" acromegaly have their HGH reduced to 10 ng/ml or less. Furthermore, in such patients the oral glucose tolerance test is likewise restored to normal, except in some patients with a family history of diabetes mellitus.

Seizures.   The classic monograph on acromegaly by Davidoff[11] listed seizures in 7 of his 100 patients. Presumably, most cases represented parasellar extensions of tumor into the temporal lobe. This complication is much less frequently encountered in current practice because patients now seek medical evaluation at an earlier stage of their disease, and the prospect that the physician will correctly appraise the problem and set the course of therapy is quite high. Following frontal craniotomy, anticonvulsants are routinely employed. We have had 1 instance of Dilantin intoxication as a result of this practice. We have had no instance of a major (grand mal) seizure by any of the methods employed, but 4 instances of mild, minor seizures have been noted in acromegalic patients following proton hypophysectomy.

Therapeutic Goals

A proposal to restate the therapeutic goals in patients harboring pituitary tumors may seem superfluous. However, amidst the profusion of clinical expressions of pituitary lesions, the exquisite panoply of laboratory tests to define the biochemical status, and the rich technology available for the therapy of pituitary tumors, the relatively simple goals of the patient may be obscured. Each patient desires safe, simple, and reliable restoration to normal health at minimal expense of personal and financial resources. The differing clinical conditions associated with pituitary tumors have different requirements.

Most patients with acromegaly simply require a reduction in circulating HGH. In addition to improvement of glucose metabolism and cessation of acral growth, it is probably more important that the eventual metabolic disabilities of acromegaly be avoided. Crippling osteoarthritis and life-threatening hypertension or cardiomyopathy are often irreversible. Since the hyperfunctioning adenoma causes visual disturbance relatively infrequently, it is undesirable to invoke a therapy that carries such a risk. When visual impairment is the presenting feature, early decompression of the optic nerves is essential. Pituitary overproduction should be curtailed, preferably without inducing hypofunction. Surgical resection by either the transfrontal or transsphenoidal routes can reduce HGH to less than 5 ng/ml. However, this normally requires total hypophysectomy and the lifelong obligations of replacement medication.

The needs in patients with Cushing's disease are similar to those in patients with acromegaly, namely, correction of the hormone excess due to hyperfunction of the pituitary. The Vanderbilt study indicates a cure of 10 of 51 patients and improvement in 13 patients by conventional x-ray alone.[12] Other therapies were applied in many of the remainder. Total adrenalectomy is probably the most widely used therapy for Cushing's disease, but it uniformly requires lifelong dependence upon corticosteroid replacement. The number of these patients who go on to develop Nelson's Syndrome seems to be increasing.[13-15] This fact together with Cushing's early demonstration of "microadenomas" in his cases[16] and with the Columbia series on pathologic findings in the pituitary,[17] is, in our view, adequate basis for including Cushing's disease of pituitary origin under the rubric of pituitary tumors. Subtotal adrenalectomy often fails to provide adequate corticosteroid reserve, and the adrenal remnant may hypertrophy to allow recurrence of Cushing's disease. Open surgical hypophysectomy has been applied with surprising rarity.

Nonfunctioning chromophobe adenomas need to be appraised in a somewhat different context. The usual symptom associated with these is visual field defect. Our present view is that chiasmal compression requires open surgery, preferably by the transsphenoidal route. Frontal craniotomy is followed by recurrence in 22% of patients unless x-ray is given, in which case the recurrence rate is reduced to 8%.[2] We are unaware of any patient preoperatively exhibiting a requirement for full maintenance of cortisone and thyroid who was restored to normal function by any method of therapy. Consequently, we do not consider restoration of normal function a feasible clinical goal in these patients.

More recently, we have treated a group of patients exhibiting an enlarged sella, no suprasellar extension of the tumor, and normal visual and endocrine functions. We have conducted Bragg peak proton radiation in them at about one-half of the dose we use in hyperfunction since our therapeutic objective is to produce only growth arrest and not necrosis. No complications have occurred since 1964. In addition, we have given proton radiation to the sella in several patients following an open surgical operation on a chromophobe adenoma.

The problem of malignant change in pituitary adenomas is particularly difficult. We understand that the histologic criteria are remarkably unreliable.[18] The cellular character of malignant pituitary tumors is often indistinguishable from the usual benign tumor. Jefferson and others have considered tumors malignant when they invade surrounding structures independent of their cytoarchitecture.[19] Implants near the pituitary may be observed. Invasion and rapid growth can occur in tumors of long duration, suggesting that change to malignancy may occur late in the course of a previously benign lesion.

One problem is to develop a diagnostic method for identifying malignant growth potential independent of histologic character. It would then be more readily possible to state whether a "cure" of a malignant tumor had been achieved. Under the present circumstances, we can only be certain of our failures.

Craniopharyngiomas, meningiomas, and various other neoplasms occur with sufficiently low frequency that they require management on an individual basis. We do advocate microsurgical technique in dealing with such lesions.

SOLUTIONS

Case Selection

Our method of case selection is rather simple. We always use the Bragg peak proton method in any instance without suprasellar extension and without excessive prior radiation exposure. If a candidate for therapy has been radiated within the previous 2 years, we allow 24 months to elapse, or we perform transsphenoidal hypophysectomy. If a patient has had more than 6000 rads of x-ray at any time in the past, we do not use protons. If he has had a full course of radiation, less than 6000 rads, more than 24 months previously, we use protons and reduce our dose by 1000–2000 rads.

If a patient has suprasellar extension, we do a transsphenoidal hypophysectomy unless the suprasellar portion is too large or is dumbbell-shaped. During transsphenoidal hypophysectomy, the dome of the tumor will usually descend as the sella is evacuated. When the distance between the tuberculum and posterior clinoids is short, the tumor is impacted and will not descend and thus necessitates a frontal craniotomy.

Acromegaly

A program for pituitary therapy has been developed on the basis of personal experience with 259 proton-treated acromegalic patients. Our initial intention is to induce focal radionecrosis of a large proportion of the adenoma. Radioimmunoassay of HGH provides a precise documentation of this procedure. Thus, in ideal instances, an acromegalic with elevated HGH and abnormal metabolism of glucose can be cured of his metabolic abnormality and experience a cessation of bone growth, accompanied by soft-tissue regression. This is accomplished with local anesthesia and with less than 2 hours on an operating table. Convalescence is uneventful. The hospital bill may be one-third to one-half the amount of that for open intracranial procedures. The patient retains normal pituitary function.

The effect of Bragg peak proton hypophysectomy on the HGH levels and clinical features of acromegaly is shown in Fig. 3. The postoperative HGH is listed in relation to the postoperative interval. The data points themselves are recorded as four grades of results on clinical criteria normally supplied by the referring physician. The solid black dots are graded "Remission" and represent reversal of all clinical indications of acromegaly—digits and facial features reduce in size, glucose intolerance normalizes, and various individual manifestations such as fatigability, sweating, joint pain, or carpal tunnel syndrome subside. Nearly all the cases falling to or below 10 ng/ml are in this grade, and this accounts for 56% of all the patients on whom we have data.

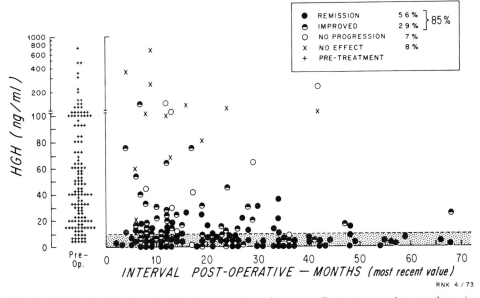

Fig. 3. HGH and clinical results following proton hypophysectomy. Posttreatment values are shown in relation to the interval postoperative in months. In each instance a single most recent value is shown. The data points indicate the degree of clinical response as shown in the box at the top right.

Furthermore, many of these patients have values 10% or less of their preoperative HGH values.

There are several instances of patients we graded clinically as "Remission" with HGH levels above 10 ng/ml, but these usually developed a fall to 30% or less of their preoperative values. We believe careful appraisal of the clinical findings and their correlation with HGH values is of major importance. In Fig. 3 we have recorded the most recent values we have for each patient with respect to the interval following therapy. Many of the values are less than 2 years postoperative and further lowering of the HGH is anticipated. We are inclined to regard the value of HGH at 2 years postoperative as the final effect, but we are aware of further decrease in HGH in some cases.

Patients who exhibit reversal of some, but not all, of the features of active acromegaly are graded as "Improved" and are represented on the figure as half-filled circles. These two grades, remission and improved, represent 85% of the patients.

The third grade, "Arrested," is represented as open circles. Seven percent of the patients fall in this group and are considered as failures in the sense that the clinical signs of acromegaly persist. This degree of response is comparable to that reported following conventional x-ray therapy.[7, 8]

Eight percent of our patients, noted by Xs, were frank "failures." They persisted in having clinical signs of active disease, and, as might be expected, their growth hormones remained high in absolute value and increased in comparison to preoperative levels. Further treatment was indicated in these patients and was provided by surgery when circumstances allowed. In general, our failures have reduced with added experience (Fig. 4).

Mortality risk in acromegalic patients is zero. Morbidity has been generally low, and in recent years, further reduced as technical resources and experience with a new method improved (Fig. 5). As is the case with most forms of pituitary ablations, it can

Cases Number	Remission	Improvement	No Progression	Failure	No Follow-up
1–50	26	16	2	6	0
51–100	27	10	3	4	6
101–150	22	14	3	2	9
151–200	17	13	5	3	12
Total	92	53	13	15	27
	145				

11/15/72 R.N.K.

Fig. 4. Proton hypophysectomy—acromegaly—results of therapy.

Cases Number	Temporary EOM Disturbance	Visual	Hypopituitary			Seizures	Retreatment
			Partial Anterior	Total Anterior	Transient D.I.		
1-50	16	3	1	7	0	0	4
51-100	14	0	0	6	1	2	4
101-150	9	1	2	3	1	1	2
151-200	3	1	1	3	2	1	3
Total	42	5	4	19	4	4	13

11/15/72 R.N.K.

Fig. 5.   Proton hypophysectomy—acromegaly—undesirable effects.

be anticipated that the morbidity is related to structures in the immediate vicinity of the pituitary.

Two factors contribute to successful application of the Bragg peak proton beam. The exact spacial distribution of the radiation must be known and controllable. Secondly, the exact spacial distribution of the pituitary and surrounding structures must be established without direct invasion of the region by the operator. Precise definition of the spacial distribution of the proton radiation was achieved by a member of the Harvard Physics Department, Mr. Andreas Koehler. A silicon diode radiation detector of $\frac{1}{4}$ mm^2 cross section sensitive area is used and the single beam of protons is carefully mapped in three dimensions. A computer program was designed to assemble a family of isodose curves of various dimensions, such that predictably high doses (up to 15,000 rads) may be developed while allowing low doses a few millimeters away. In general the dose falls off from the central high-intensity region at the rate of 1000–2000 rads/mm (Fig. 6).

It is mandatory to secure radiographically precise measurements of the pituitary area in each individual patient. Several necessary studies have evolved with the aid of our neuroradiological colleagues, Dr. Taveras, Dr. New, and Dr. Roberson. Since all x-ray films are secured with more or less enlargement of the skeletal or contrast images, it is necessary to correct for such magnification. We secure marker films taken with leadshot markers at intervals of 10 mm placed in the three planes of the pituitary —midline, coronal, and horizontal (to Reed's line). Pneumoencephalography is used to evaluate regions above the clinoids. It is imperative to determine whether suprasellar extension of the tumor exists, for such cases are ordinarily excluded from proton beam therapy. In addition, the course of the optic nerves can be established from the recesses of the third ventricle and the details of the optic cistern, in part, with the aid of tomography. Coronal polytomes of the floor of the sella are very helpful. During the past year, cavernous sinography has been routinely employed to provide additional precise measurement of the internal limits of the tumor.

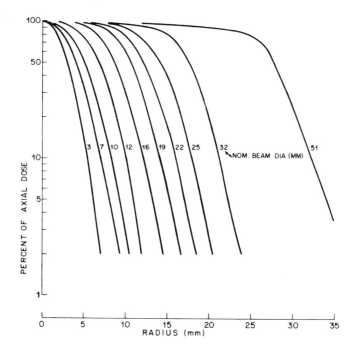

Fig. 6.   Radial dose distributions at the proton Bragg peak at a depth of 11 cm in water. Our convention is to state the total dose in terms of the axial dose. This dose falls along radii from the axis depending upon the beam diameter. Note that although the rate of fall of the dose below about 70% of the axial dose is linear on the graph, the vertical scale is logarithmic.

We have had 2 optic nerve complications (1 hemianopsia and 1 quadrantanopsia) since a new dosimetry has been employed (after case No. 100). In 2 other patients in whom x-radiation had been used prior to proton radiation, field defects developed. The risk to optic nerves in patients who have previously received x-ray therapy is about two times as great as in those without prior radiation exposure. Visual loss in association with the so-called "empty sella syndrome" is, in part, associated with whatever therapy is employed, and it accrued in 2 patients. Two patients developed visual loss postoperatively due to diabetic retinopathy, and another patient had a visual defect due to an arachnoid cyst of the middle fossa and chiasmatic cistern. There have been no field defects since 1971 in 72 acromegalic patients.

Temporary Oculomotor Disturbance.   This has been the most persistent problem. Many patients are aware of the problem only intermittently upon waking, turning, changing gaze, or when fatigued. In others the eye casts out or ptosis may occur. The disturbance recovers in a variable number of months. In 1 patient a second course of radiation was followed by diplopia, which has persisted 55 months and is evidently permanent. Another patient has worn an eye patch continuously, and her diplopia has persisted. The frequency of this problem has decreased with the technical maneuvers described below.

In our early experience, instances of transient oculomotor disturbance occurred with a significant frequency (Fig. 5). This figure shows a substantial reduction with improved dosimetry and other technical refinements. The high-dose radiation was moved 1 mm medially to the perimeter of pituitary tissue in the anticipation that the outermost zone should be normal gland rather than adenoma. In addition, by moving the center of rotation of the radiation pattern 5 mm beyond the midline, the beams passing through the cavernous sinus are more divergent, and the radiation to these nerves attributable to overlap of beams is reduced.

The decrement in frequency of oculomotor complications in cases No. 101–200 does not include the anticipated advantage from cavernous sinography. In the past 96 cases in 3 years, the only oculomotor disturbance occurred in a neurotic female with apparent invasion of her cavernous sinus. The oculomotor nerves range between 2 and 7 mm lateral to the pituitary. Thus, nerves that are closest to the pituitary are at greater risk than those further away laterally. In the sinograms, the lateral walls of the pituitary are evident, but the individual oculomotor nerves cannot be identified.

Hypopituitarism. We consider hypofunction of the pituitary an undesirable effect. The majority of the patients treated by the Bragg peak proton method retain normal pituitary function. We noted hypofunction in 27 cases of 231 acromegalics treated by November, 1972 (Fig. 5) by the proton beam. The requirement for cortisone and thyroid was present in 19 patients. An additional 4 patients required either thyroid or cortisone but not both. In addition we have identified HGH deficiency in 5 patients with HGH values below 1 ng/ml who fail to respond to insulin or arginine stimulation and develop reactive hypoglycemia late in a glucose tolerance test. Four patients had transient diabetes insipidus.

Seizures. We have been concerned from our beginning with Bragg peak proton therapy that the dose of radiation to the medial temporal lobe may be significant. In collaboration with pathologists, we studied the brains of 8 patients who had received proton radiation by our original technique.[20] These patients had all been irradiated with the beam portals in a single horizontal plane (since at that time we did not have the resources to compute isodose curves in a three-dimensional system). Although none of these patients exhibited appropriate clinical symptoms, several of the medial temporal regions show changes regarded as consistent with radiation effects a few millimeters in size. Our concern over this matter had induced us to modify the arrangement of portals prior to the time this study was completed so that the portals diverged vertically as well as horizontally. No instance of histologic change has been seen since.

Cushing's Disease

The principles evolved in the treatment of acromegaly are all directly applicable to Cushing's disease due to pituitary ACTH excess. A radiographically normal sella is found in fewer cases of acromegaly (about 5%) than in Cushing's disease. (This figure is not well established for Cushing's disease, but in our experience, at least 30% ultimately develop abnormal sellae.)

Nevertheless, the principles and techniques of hypophysectomy by the Bragg peak proton method are identical. The results are quite similar (Figs. 7*a* and 7*b*). We have treated 56 patients. We can report followup on 43 of them. Eighty-nine percent are improved, including 58% with complete remission. Seven patients with sustained high levels of cortisol or who required additional therapy were rated as failures (11%).

	HYPERCORTICISM	NELSON'S SYNDROME	TOTAL
Remission	27	3	30
Improved	2	4	6
Failed	7	0	7
Incomplete	12	1	13
TOTAL	48	8	56

7-31-73 RNK

(a)

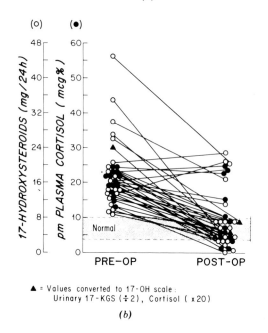

▲ = Values converted to 17-OH scale :
Urinary 17-KGS (÷2), Cortisol (x20)

(b)

Fig. 7. (a) Proton hypophysectomy—Cushing's disease—results of therapy. Both hypercorticoid patients and those with Nelson's syndrome—pituitary tumor and hyperpigmentation are included in data. (b) Corticosteroid values in patients with hypercorticism before and after proton beam. Steroid values are given for 36 patients with hypercorticism. Most of these values are in terms of urinary 17-hydroxy steroids or plasma cortisols adjusted to a comparable scale. In a few instances, only urinary 17-ketogenic steroids or urinary cortisols were available and were converted to scale according to the conversion factors indicated.

Whether or not the patient has had prior adrenal surgery has little influence on the prospect or interval to achieve a remission. However, in a few instances of early or mild Cushing's Disease, a good response has been evident in only 1 month following therapy. The ideal result is superior to that experienced in acromegalic patients since all the stigmata of the condition may be obliterated.

Complications have been mild and infrequent, and they follow the pattern of those seen in the acromegalic patients (Fig. 8). They are: 1 unilateral quadrantanopsia (1969), 4 instances of temporary oculomotor disturbance, and 3 cases of hypopituitarism. One patient underwent at approximately 2-year intervals, x-ray, proton beam, transsphenoidal hypophysectomy, and bilateral total adrenalectomy. Her adrenals showed multinodularity with a large hyperplastic nodule thought to be autonomous. She did poorly after her adrenalectomy and died of a stroke but was not autopsied.

Chromophobe Adenoma

Risk to the optic nerves is avoided by identifying in a pneumoencephalogram the absence of tumor above the clinoids and tracing the course of the optic nerves from the chiasm between the suprachiasmatic and suprapituitary recesses to their entrance into the optic foramina just below the level of the tuberculum of the sphenoid.

Patients with suprasellar extension require open surgical hypophysectomy, for which we prefer the transsphenoidal route because none of our patients treated in this manner have experienced a fatality, nor have they experienced the emergence or aggravation of a field defect. We line the cavity with gold foil and follow the patients with periodic x-rays to detect shifts of the gold foil and with visual fields examinations.

Retreatment can be done by any of several methods. We do not know the reoperation rate for the transsphenoidal operation in the larger series. In some centers, conventional x-ray is given routinely immediately postoperative. Ray et al as mentioned, had a recurrence rate of 8% in transfrontally operated patients who received postoperative x-ray. We consider it to be a liability if it is necessary to x-irradiate all patients for the

	Hypercorticism	Nelson's Syndrome	Total
NUMBER OF PATIENTS	44	8	52
TEMPORARY OCULOMOTOR DISTURBANCE	3	1	4
VISUAL LOSS	1	0	1
HYPOPITUITARY			
Anterior Partial	1	0	1
Anterior Total	2	0	2
Posterior Temporary	0	0	0
Posterior Permanent	0	0	0
Retreatment	5	0	5

11/15/72 R.N.K.

Fig. 8.   Proton hypophysectomy—Cushing's disease—undesirable effects.

limited gain of reducing the recurrence rate from 22 to 8% Thus, only 14% are really benefitted, while 100% are subject to the expense, inconvenience, and income loss that is associated with a course of x-ray therapy.

Of 46 patients treated since 1964 by the proton beam for benign chromophobe adenoma, to date, 1 has been known to develop a recurrence of solid tumor, and transsphenoidal hypophysectomy was done. We operated on 2 other patients with developing field defects by the transsphenoidal route and found fluid-filled cysts, 1 with a tan layer on the walls and the other with glistening white fibrous tissue on its walls. Pathologic examination confirmed no recurrence in the cyst walls.

It is considered that therapy of asymptomatic nonfunctioning adenomas will prevent the progress of these lesions to chiasmal compression. It is probably better to employ the minimal risk of limited dose radiation therapy than to deal with the chiasmal syndrome by craniotomy at a later date. The custom of serial plain skull x-rays and visual field examinations does little to protect the patient from the development of a suprasellar extension of the tumor.

Patients with Forbes-Albright syndrome, amenorrhea/galactorrhea, are now known to have elevated levels of prolactin. We do not have follow-up prolactin levels as yet on the patients we have treated.

Malignant Chromophobe Tumors

One step in the solution of the problem of malignant pituitary tumors is to characterize them by their growth character. This can be done in tumor tissue culture. The malignant lesions we have seen have had growth rates in tissue culture several times greater than ordinary adenomas as shown by the culture methods of our colleague, Dr. Paul Kornblith.[21]

We have 3 proven cases and another possible case in our 305 proton-beam-treated acromegalic and chromophobe adenoma patients of a tumor considered benign at the time of initial proton treatment and later becoming malignant. It would be of interest to us to confirm whether or not our experience gives any statistical confidence as to whether we might have either prevented or cured malignant change in a pituitary adenoma.

AUTHOR'S METHODS

Stereotactic Bragg Peak Proton Hypophysectomy

The accelerated protons are extracted from the cyclotron by bending magnets and are concentrated into a beam by focusing magnets. Figure 9 portrays the sequence of manipulations of the proton beam. A fixed absorber reduces the initial energy to an amount that will penetrate to about 12 cm in water or an equivalent medium such as brain tissue. The particle beam next passes through holes in brass collimator plates, separated by 1 meter so that the protons emerging from the final collimator are virtually parallel in their paths and produce a beam with a sharply defined edge. The variable water absorber adjusts the depth of penetration of the Bragg peak.

Increasingly precise dosimetry has been developing through the work of our physicist colleagues during the life of this program. An integrating ion dosimeter with nitrogen

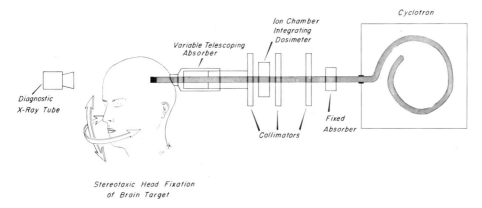

Fig. 9.   Diagram of the sequence in the course of a proton beam from acceleration to cranial target. The diagram indicates the basic relation between the principal components of the system.

chamber measures the radiation passing through it. Prior to therapeutic exposure of a patient, the nitrogen-chamber dosimeter is calibrated against the absolute standard of a Faraday cup which collects all the radiation emerging from the final collimator. The Faraday cup is in the place of the patient's head shown in Fig. 9. Detailed point by point measurement of the beam is made possible by a silicon diode detector that was developed by one of our physics staff.[22] The tiny dosimeter with a cross section sensitive area of $\frac{1}{4}$ mm^2 has been used to map the beams of various diameters.

Figure 10 shows the isodose contours of such a beam, 7 mm in diameter. The radiation to the pituitary gland is delivered through 12 portals of entry on each side of the head in three tiers. The computations of the three-dimensional isodose curve for one

DOSE IN PERCENT OF PEAK DOSE
7mm DIAM. BEAM WITH ~12.5 cm RANGE

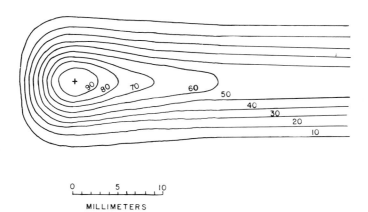

Fig. 10.   Isodose curve of a single proton beam. The cross section of the beam through its central axis is mapped in three dimensions by a silicon diode radiation detector with a sensitive area of $\frac{1}{4}$ mm.^{2}

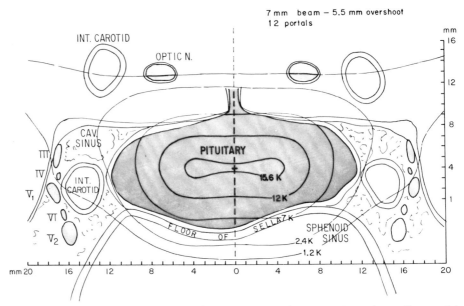

Fig. 11.   Computer-produced isodose curve of twelve converging beams superimposed on a diagram of the pituitary region. Isodose curves are a three-dimension composite determined by a computer for beams of various diameters and for various widths of the pituitary fossa.

central coronal plane is done by a computer, as shown in Fig. 11. The sizes of the portals, their configuration, and the radiation dose is altered for specific situations.

For the radiation of pituitary tumors, portals up to 25 mm in diameter have been used. Normally, fewer portals are used in very large targets. To induce frank radionecrosis in most pituitary targets (except chromophobe adenoma), large doses of 6000–10,000 rads at the Bragg peak are used. When the object of therapy is to induce growth arrest of chromophobe adenoma, the dose is 2000–4000 rads. The dose at the site of entrance and along the path of a single beam is about one-twentieth that of the central target dose. Figure 12 is an example in which 7000 rads is delivered to the pituitary

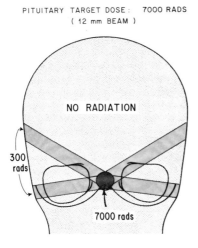

Fig. 12.   Example of proton radiation dose and distribution in the coronal plane. The diagram represents an approximately coronal plane of the head through the pituitary target, taken from the protocol of a typical patient with acromegaly. Four of the 12 entering beams are shown; the remainder are anterior or posterior to this plane. The small dose of radiation along the beam path and the absence of radiation throughout most of the brain is indicated. The pituitary target dose is ample to induce radionecrosis confined to the pituitary.

with a 12 mm beam. In this example the dose to the temporal lobe along the beam path is 300 rads, and the remaining temporal lobe and cerebrum receive essentially no radiation (less than 1 rad).

In our method, the entire course of radiation is completed in 30–40 minutes. This dose rate is roughly 1500 times as great as that normally employed in conventional x-ray.

The stereotactic instrument as shown in Fig. 13 is a modification of our general-purpose stereotactic instrument.[23] The instrument has two axes of rotation, a vertical one and a horizontal one, about which the instrument, fixed to the patient's head, may rotate. The instrument allows the head to be adjusted in three planes so that the pituitary or other target is located just exactly on these two axes of rotation. The Bragg peak of the proton beam is directed to the exact intersection of these two axes and, therefore, to the pituitary target.

To illustrate the method, Fig. 14 shows radiographic confirmation of this superimposition of the proton beam upon the pituitary (a small circle and a central dot on the radiograph marked by a beam spot in the pituitary fossa). Alignment of the beam is

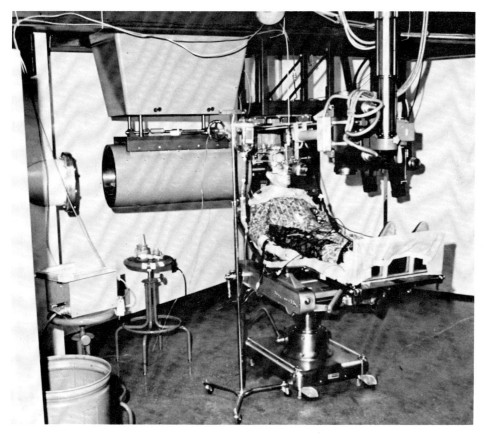

Fig. 13. Patient in stereotactic instrument undergoing proton radiation. The patient's head affixed to the stereotaxic instrument is seen in the center. Left: the system of collimators and the ion chamber is housed in a large cylinder; far left: the source of the beam from the cyclotron; right: diagnostic x-ray equipment for centering the pituitary target.

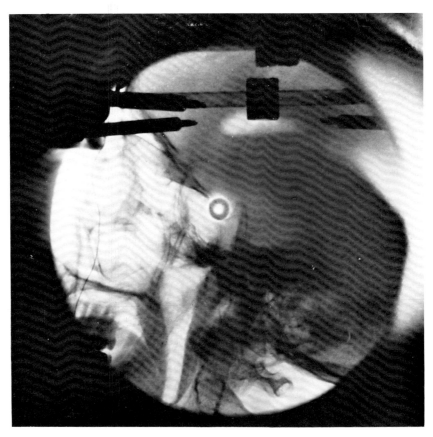

Fig. 14. Beam spot—exposure of protons on a radiograph of sella turcica. A skull x-ray taken during the alignment of the proton beam with the pituitary target shows the brief exposure of the proton beam exposed on the x-ray film—the "beam spot."

precisely confirmed by Polaroid radiographs before the therapeutic exposure is performed.

Depth of penetration of the Bragg peak is controlled by the variable water absorber (Fig. 9) which automatically corrects for various differences in the length of the path through the head at the various portal sites. Computed corrections in length of the path are introduced to account for variations in radiation absorption by the bone and tissues. Six portals, vertically displaced in three banks on each side of the head, are normally delivered in about 40 minutes.

A beam diameter is selected appropriate to the dimensions of the sella. From the pneumoencephalogram we determine the course of the optic nerve. The center of the beam is brought to lie a distance below the plane of the optic nerves so that they receive not more than 1000 rads. Figure 6 displays the radial dose distribution for beams of several sizes from which we establish the radiation dose at any particular point. The beam center is placed 2 mm anteriorly to the midpoint of the sella to spare the posterior lobe from high doses of radiation. In patients with acromegaly and Cushing's disease, the beam diameter is selected to leave a 1 mm shell around the margins of the sella, since this usually is the remnant of normal pituitary gland, and normal pituitary function may thus be preserved.

The entire therapeutic procedure is done in a single stage or sitting, under local anesthesia, in usually 1½ hours. The patient walks to and from the procedure at the Harvard cyclotron, walks away from it, leaves the hospital in 2 days, and can immediately return to home and occupation.

Measurable decrease in pituitary or end-organ hormones may be detected 1–6 months following the procedure. It is considered stabilized 1–2 years later, at which time the values obtained are considered as the ultimate result of the therapy.

Microsurgical Transsphenoidal Hypophysectomy

We learned of Guiot's method over 10 years ago and have been gratified to see its development in North America by Hardy. On their precedent we use an operating microscope, a Zeiss double binocular microscope. We use a Siemens image amplifier for both fluoroscopy and films that is oriented for lateral viewing. We open the anterior wall of the sphenoid widely and aspirate, resect, and curette all the contents of the sella turcica. Normally the diaphragm and the arachnoid can be maintained intact without provoking free flow of cerebrospinal fluid, although pinhole openings may occur. A bundle representing the pituitary stalk is normally apparent, and we leave a few millimeters of this structure because we believe the maneuver minimizes the usual brief episode of postoperative diabetes insipidus.

We normally line the cavity with multiple folded segments of gold foil placed against the diaphragm, cavernous sinus, and bony boundaries. These markers have proved to be useful in follow-up evaluation for the question of recurrence. We have adopted the policy of not conducting postoperative radiation on a routine basis. Instead the patients are followed with periodic radiographic examinations wherein we compare the gold foil contour and position with that obtained shortly after the operation. We anticipate that shifts in the foil would be evidence of recurrence and radiation would then be performed.

We normally secure a segment of fascia lata to line the superior and the anterior surfaces of the sella. If the fascia is slack, we introduce a bit of fat taken at the same time to support the fascia against these surfaces. A piece of nasal cartilage is wedged into the defect in the anterior wall. The sphenoid and nasal cavities are packed with finger cots and condoms loosely filled with Bacitracin-soaked gauze and lubricated with Bacitracin Ointment. Antibiotics are given by injection. Packs are gradually removed on the third to fifth day.

Microsurgical Transfrontal Hypophysectomy

We began using the operating microscope for pituitary surgery in 1963 and later included the image amplifier in much the same manner as described above for transsphenoidal surgery. We open a right frontal bone flap for symmetric tumors. If the tumor is asymmetric, we open the side contralateral to the highest portion because it is easier to deal with the large mass by traversing the sella diagonally. We seek to minimize traction and elevation of the frontal lobe and expose only the lower portion of the tumor presenting between the optic nerves. We seek scrupulously to preserve the blood vessels on the superior surface. Bergland and Ray drew attention to the importance of this blood supply nourishing the optic chiasm.[24] As the tumor is evacuated, the dome can be drawn down into the field. In the final stages, the surface of the dome can be mobilized sufficiently to remove remnants of tumor from its undersurface. The contents of the sella are evacuated and curetted. Occasionally, a tiny mirror is useful in visualizing the depths of the sella. The image amplifier is used during final curettage to assure that the curettage is thorough on the floor and anterior wall. Gold foil is placed on the floor and the lateral walls. The image amplifier confirms that the foil is applied closely to the bony outlines and that no gaps representing tumor are remaining. Gold foil is also placed against the diaphragm, and the postoperative x-rays are as shown in Fig. 15. Again, these x-ray records have the dual purpose of checking for any suspicion of postoperative hemorrhage and for later periodic appraisal of possible recurrence. Postoperative antibiotics are not given unless the frontal sinus is opened.

DISCUSSION

The system of surgery described herein for pituitary tumors appears to have virtually eliminated the risk of mortality associated with therapeutic procedures except for those risks associated with use of general anesthesia, such as pulmonary embolism and hepatitis. The overall morbidity is low, largely attributable to the preponderance of proton-treated cases.

The patients' acceptance of the proton procedure under only local anesthesia is quite good. Their attitude and emotional preparation is largely attributable to the fact that

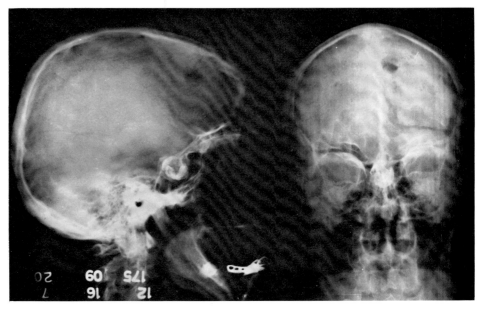

Fig. 15. X-Rays showing folded layers of gold foil lining the sella turcica. Gold foil is folded in several layers and matted against the inner boundaries of the pituitary tumor after it has been excised. Follow-up x-ray examinations can be compared to detect shifts in the foil, which would be early evidence of tumor recurrence.

all the members of the clinical team—endocrinologist, surgeon, nurse, and anesthetist, spend ample amounts of time explaining the procedure and answering their questions. They are, in general, comfortable and reassured during the 1½–2 hour period of the stereotactic procedure.

The hospital costs associated with proton therapy compare well with the other methods in these patients, as shown in Fig. 16. The expense of frontal craniotomy is about three times as great as that of proton hypophysectomy, and transsphenoidal hypophysectomy is midway between these. This is largely attributable to the difference in length of hospital stay following a procedure, as shown in Fig. 17. In addition to the short in-hospital convalescence, there is no home convalescence of work disability. In the past it has not been the custom to consider costs in a clinical or scientific paper. Times are changing, however, and we are all increasingly aware of the influences outside of medical practice (third parties, government) whereby cost is a major determinant of policy. Physicians should consider this matter or lose initiative in formulation of policies relating to medical care.

Partly because of the escalation of medical costs, the cost of air travel to the cyclotron from mid-North America is approximately equivalent to the cost of 1 day of hospitalization. Thus, two cyclotrons in the United States are ample for the national needs of such a resource. A multiplication of medical cyclotrons would make them all prohibitively inefficient unless substantial expansion of cyclotron applications were to occur.

We presume it to be the intent of this symposium to allow comparisons to be made between the many alternatives available in diagnosis and management of pituitary tumors. Because of the difficulty in making worthwhile comparisons between nonstandardized format and definitions employed by various workers, we recommend that uniform standards for evaluation of methods and results be formulated for systems of pituitary therapy. This is another instance in which physicians should exercise initiative before they find others doing it for them. Unwarranted mortality, morbidity, and expense may well become of interest to peer review committees and government in the coming decade.

| | OPEN | | Bragg Peak Proton Beam Hypophysectomy |
	Frontal Craniotomy	Transsphenoidal Hypophysectomy	
AVERAGE	$5,005	$2,713	$1,569
MINIMUM	$4,227	$2,338	$ 855
MAXIMUM	$6,501	$3,154	$2,391

11/15/72-R.N.K.

Fig. 16. Surgical treatment methods—comparison of hospital costs.

DIAGNOSIS	OPEN Frontal Craniotomy	OPEN Transsphenoidal	Bragg Peak Proton Beam Hypophysectomy
ACROMEGALY	18	10	2
CUSHING'S DISEASE	17	16	2
CHROMOPHOBE ADENOMA	16	18	2
OTHER	14	20	3

11/15/72-R.N.K.

Fig. 17.   Hospital days—Procedure to discharge.

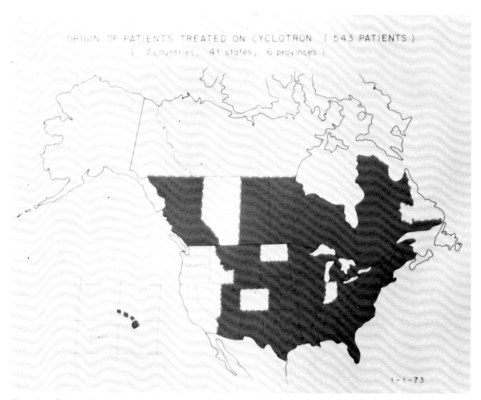

Fig. 18.   Origin of patients treated on cyclotron (543 patients).

The management of pituitary tumors tends to be more or less a function of "centers." An epidemiologist tells us that there are about 2500 newly diagnosed pituitary tumors each year in the United States or a bit over 1 per year per neurosurgeon.[25] Inevitably, most of the pituitary surgery will be performed by a limited number of neurosurgeons. The epidemiologist further reports that only about 300 new cases of acromegaly emerge each year. On this basis, between the Berkeley cyclotron and ourselves, about half of the new cases of acromegaly are currently being treated by particle radiation beams.[26]

We are grateful to the physicians who have permitted us to work in this fascinating area. Our cases are usually fully evaluated by referring endocrinologists, frequently from endocrine units of university hospitals spread widely over the United States and Canada (Fig. 18). In many instances the referral is accompanied by a pneumoencephalogram and test results for the major pituitary functions. A detailed endocrine and physiologic survey is completed during the same time required for the further radiodiagnostic procedures. Visual acuity and perimetry is obtained immediately prior to the treatment procedure. Patients return to their referring physicians, who have been extraordinarily helpful in providing follow-up evaluation and data. We have recommended extensive follow-up at 6, 12, and 24 months, with an annual follow-up thereafter. This approach has provided the most useful information as to the reliability of treatment techniques and secures a high degree of medical observation and care for every patient.

ACKNOWLEDGMENTS

Dr. Bernard Kliman, Endocrine Unit, Massachusetts General Hospital, has been a full collaborator in this work. He has conducted pretreatment and posttreatment evaluation on these patients and assisted in the preparation of this material. The author gratefully acknowledges the theoretical and technical services of the cyclotron crew of the Harvard Physics Department, particularly Mr. Andreas M. Koehler and Dr. William M. Preston. I thank the nurses and technicians of the Endocrine Unit and Laboratory. I especially thank Dr. William H. Sweet, Chief of Neurosurgery, and Dr. Alexander Leaf, Chief of Medicine, Massachusetts General Hospital, for counsel and support. I particularly thank Miss Rita Thompson and Mrs. Billie Swisher for the compilation of data and editorial work.

REFERENCES

1. Henderson, W. R.: The Pituitary Adenomata. A Follow-up Study of the Surgical Results in 338 Cases (Dr. Harvey Cushing's series). *Brit. J. Surg.* **26**:811–921 (1939).

2. Ray, B. S., and Patterson, R. H.: Surgical Experience with Chromophobe Adenomas of the Pituitary Gland. *J. Neurosurg.* **34**:726–729 (1971).

3. Ray, B. S., Horwith, M., and Mautalen, C.: Surgical Hypophysectomy as a Treatment for Acromegaly. In Astwood, E. B., and Cassidy, C. E., Eds., *Clinical Endocrinology. II*, Grune & Stratton, New York, 1968, pp. 93–102.

4. Hamlin, H.: Personal communications, 1971.

5. Lee, W. M. and Adams, J. E.: The Empty Sella Syndrome. *J. Neurosurg.* **28**:351–356 (1968).

6. Kjellberg, R. N., Shintani, A., Frantz, A. G., and Kliman, B.: Proton Beam Therapy in Acromegaly. *New Engl. J. Med.* **278**:689–695 (1968).

7. Glick, S. M.: Clinical Staff Conference. Acromegaly and Other Disorders of Growth Hormone Secretion: Combined Clinical Staff Conference at National Institutes of Health. *Ann. Internal Med.* **66**:760–788 (1967).

8. Roth, J., Gorden, P., and Brace, K.: Efficacy of Conventional Pituitary Irradiation in Acromegaly. *New Engl. J. Med.* **282:**1385–1391 (1970)

9. Adams, J. E., Seymour, R. J. Earl, J. M., Tuele, M., Sparks, L. L., and Forsham, P. H.: Transsphenoidal Cryohypophysectomy in Acromegaly, Clinical and Endocrinological Evaluation. *J. Neurosurg.* **28:**100–104 (1968).

10. Rand, R. W.: Cryosurgery of the Pituitary in Acromegaly: Reduced Growth Hormone Levels Following Hypophysectomy in 13 Cases. *Ann. Surg.* **164:**587–592 (1966).

11. Davidoff, L. M.: Studies in Acromegaly. III. The Anamnesis and Symptomatology in One Hundred Cases. *Endocrinology* **10:**461–483 (1926).

12. Orth, D. N., and Liddle, G. W.: Results of Treatment in 108 Patients with Cushing's Syndrome. *New Engl. J. Med.* **285:**243–247 (1971).

13. Sprague, R. G., Weeks, R. E., Priestley, J. T., and Salassa, R. M.: Treatment of Cushing's Syndrome by Adrenalectomy. In Gardiner-Hill, H., Ed., *Modern Trends in Endocrinology,* Paul B. Hoeber, New York, 1961, pp. 84–99.

14. Salassa, R. M., Kearns, T. P., Kernohan, J. W., Sprague, R. G., and MacCarty, C. S.: Pituitary Tumors in Patients with Cushing's Syndrome. *J. Clin. Endocrinol.* **19:**1523–1539 (1959).

15. Randall, R. V.: Personal communication, 1973.

16. Cushing, H.: The Basophil Adenomas of the Pituitary Body and their Clinical Manifestations (pituitary basophilism). *Bull. Johns Hopkins Hosp.* **50:**137–195 (1932).

17. Plotz, C. M., Knowlton, A. I., and Ragan, C.: Natural History of Cushing's Syndrome. *Amer. J. Med.* **13:**597–614 (1952).

18. Russfield, A. B.: Diseases of the Pituitary. In Minckler, J., Ed., *Pathology of the Nervous System. I.,* McGraw-Hill, New York, 1968, pp. 619–638.

19. Jefferson, G.: Extrasellar Extensions of Pituitary Adenomas. In *Sir Geoffrey Jefferson: Selected Papers,* Charles C Thomas, Illinois, 1960, p. 375.

20. Nielsen, S. L., Kjellberg, R. N., Asbury, A. K., and Koehler, A. M.: Neuropathologic Effects of Proton-Beam Irradiation in Man. II. Evaluation after Pituitary Irradiation. *Acta. Neuropathol.* **21:**76–82 (1972).

21. Kornblith, P. L.: Personal communication, 1973.

22. Koehler, A. M.: Dosimetry of Proton Beams Using Small Silicon Diodes. *Rad. Res. Suppl.* **7:**53–63 (1967).

23. Kjellberg, R. N., Koehler, A. M., Preston, W. M., and Sweet, W. H.: Stereotaxic Instrument for Use with the Bragg Peak of a Proton Beam. *Confina Neurol.* **22:**183–189 (1962).

24. Bergland, R., and Ray, B. S.: The Arterial Supply of the Human Optic Chiasm. *J. Neurosurg.* **31:**327–334 (1969).

25. Poskanzer, D. C.: Personal communication, 1972.

26. Lawrence, J. H., Tobias, C. A. Linfoot, J. A., Born, J. L., Lyman, J. T., Chong, C. Y., Manougian, E., and Wei, W. C.: Successful Treatment of Acromegaly: Metabolic and Clinical Studies in 145 Patients. *J. Clin. Endocrinol.* **31:**180–198 (1970).

Discussion

Dr. Seydel. Thank you very much Dr. Kjellberg. Before opening the discussion I would like to ask Dr. Mullan to say a few words about surgery.

Dr. Mullan. This has been a most impressive collection of papers; Dr. Kramer's, Dr. Sheline's very impressive group of statistics and Dr. Levin's detailed analysis of the type of tumor and lastly Dr. Kjellberg's details on the proton beam. I think in particular we must not say all chromophobes must be treated this way and all acromegalics should be treated that way. The treatment for each patient must be individualized, that is, for patients with high or low growth hormone levels. Among patients with chromophobe adenoma, signs and symptoms may consist of large sellas, endocrine trouble, missed periods, loss of libido, as well as loss of vision. All of these are going to be treated somewhat differently according to the particular problem that we have to deal with. There is no representative of Dr. Hardy here but we should emphasize again the delightful results that can be obtained in a small number of discrete tumors that can pop out through the operating microscope inserted through the nose. You leave a nice gland behind and no problems. It's a small group but it's always worth considering that group. Among acromegalics one must consider if one's patient fits into this group where one can have a nice discrete removal. In the chromophobes, I think it depends really what the problem is. If the patient presents with a large sella, one has got to make sure that it's not an empty sella. Too many empty sellas have been treated by a variety of means. We have to make sure that that is not due to an aneurysm, not due to meningioma, or not due to a whole variety of the odd things we have collected over the years such as cysticercosis of the sella. You can get almost anything in the sella so one cannot just assume because of a large sella that there is a chromophobe adenoma. But what does one do if one has a patient who has a large sella and some loss of vision? My own feeling is that if one is sure that it's nothing else as well as one can by angiogram, by scan, by all the means at our disposal, and the loss of vision is limited to the upper outer quadrant, I certainly would advise radiotherapy before advising surgery. The visual defect should disappear because radiotherapy is specific for chromophobe adenomas, but if the vision does not improve with radiotherapy then I think we should look and find out what it really is. If the visual defect appears at the outer lower quadrant, then I am not so sure what to do. I have fairly strong feelings and these decisions are rather arbitrary. If the visual loss crosses the midline, it's time to relieve that surgically rather than trying radiotherapy. These are arbitrary decisions and I am sure there is no concensus of opinion at this time. I have seen patients over the years deteriorate during the course of radiotherapy and some have to come to surgery rather abruptly, sometimes after they had lost vision suddenly. Which brings us to the question of surgical mortality. We have had a number of reports of surgical mortality here, all of which are accurate, but I cannot agree with the conclusions drawn. The reports are accurate but the conclusions are not. It depends on who manages the patient. If I were to treat with Bragg peak radiation, that would be disastrous. It would be absolutely disastrous because I know nothing about the proton beam. You have to have the expert. When you treat with a transnasal approach you must remember who to treat transnasally and many of us do this. It's no great technique as far as technical difficulty is concerned, but you tend to get a group of people who are rather skillful and spend a lot of effort doing this. The average neurosurgeon doesn't operate through a microscope and the average neurosurgeon doesn't operate through the nose. The people who are operating up through the nose with a microscope are a group of particularly skilled people who spent a lot of time developing that technique and, therefore, they are experts in the field. Transfrontal treatment is not the same. An examiner of the Board of Neurosurgery found out what people have done in the 2 years after finishing training until they come up for their boards, and each candidate was supposed to keep a record of all the operations. He looked over pituitaries and he found that a group of candidates coming up for their boards 2 years after finishing their residency had a 12% mortality. That is rather poor. This is not an indictment of the transfrontal method. Again it depends who is doing it. If you have an expert doing the transfrontal method, there is no reason in the world why you should have mortality. It's the simplest of all neurosurgical procedures. If the patient cannot tolerate general anesthesia or you don't like the general anesthesiologist, you operate under local. The transfrontal operation is a simple operation but you have to work on a brain without pressure. If you try to retract the brain, of course, you are going to get into trouble. You will get postoperative epilepsy, postoperative swelling, you will get all sorts of problems. But you must know how to do it. These are not bloody tumors and there is no problem with hemostasis. So there is no reason in the world why there should be any mortality. Similarly when one is giving radiotherapy it depends who is giving it. Let's not compare transfrontal with transnasal surgery with Bragg peak radiation.

Now we come to the difficult one and I am not sure that any of us have an answer, and that is the large tumor. Dr. Kramer showed a couple of examples and I really don't know how to tackle those. Some of them are malignant. In 20 years the only patient with a pituitary I have lost is a patient who was in a coma 2 days and had a tumor growing into the frontal lobe which was frankly a malignant tumor, which penetrated the anterior substance. As I mentioned in my earlier talk the anterior substance is sacred. You cannot operate on that; it just doesn't work. Now what would I do with those two cases that you showed, and as I said before I don't know what I would do. If it was very vascular, then I think I would be worried that this was a malignant invasive tumor and I would call for a scan and ask for the exact limitations and if it seemed to be infiltrating the brain I wouldn't touch it. If it is not vascular and not a malignant one, then even though it's large I don't see there is any reason why one cannot tackle it and decompress it. I would look forward in the future more and more to the developments in nuclear imaging which will tell us precisely and exactly where the tumor is so that Dr. Kjellberg would be able to concentrate a beam on this more and more closely.

Dr. Kramer. I think Dr. Mullan has raised an extremely difficult point. Of course, it depends who does what. I think that goes for all of medicine after all, and I think what one is trying to do here is to compare in a way one expert's results with another expert's results and then see to what extent this can be applied across the country. I mean if you have a wonderful technique that will only affect one per hundred thousand of the population it's really a wonderful technique but it doesn't do the whole group of patients with that disease much good. So until we get to the point that I mentioned earlier where we can do control studies in all these areas, I don't think that particular answers can be obtained. In the meantime, we will have to continue trying to get the best results and compare them with somebody else's best results.

I think Dr. Kjellberg's paper is of great interest and the only question I would raise is it seems to me that even in his expert hands the group of patients whose growth hormone levels have been reduced is about the same as that of Dr. Sheline, and as we have shown in the group treated by conventional radiation therapy, the number of patients requiring substitutional therapy is about the same. We found that about 15 of our people required cortisone and thyroid, without surgery. So that it becomes a matter of choice as to which technique you employ. I think one will have to look over the years a little more closely at the morbidity produced to finally come to a conclusion as to which method is best.

Dr. Sheline.   Just two or three comments. I might start out with what I think should be a defense of our neurosurgeons. I think we have got a pretty good crew and you will notice I mentioned that since 1945 there have been 4 out of 88 deaths in the craniopharyngioma group, but you will note 1 of these was a cerebral infarction, a carotid artery problem, and how to explain this away I don't know. The other 3 were all in a very large and locally invasive tumor. Our pathologists have a great deal of difficulty distinguishing a malignant one from a nonmalignant one on a morphologic basis, but these were the type that invaded temporal or frontal lobes and it was in these that they had the mortality. I think perhaps my own thought here would be that perhaps simply a biopsy and a minimal amount of decompression with some radiotherapy would have been the preferable way to do it. I think this particular kind of lesion incidentally is not one suitable for proton or Bragg peak radiation because I believe you must treat large volumes and therefore I don't think there is any way on earth you can precisely delineate the extent of the tumor without doing an autopsy.

Dr. Kjellberg.   I think your figure of 12% hypopituitarism was treatment-induced hypopituitarism, not preoperative. At the same time you showed a 56% remission rate although some of these patients still had elevated growth hormone levels. I wonder if you would compare this with the Berkeley data? Either you or Dr. Levin probably knows it better than I. I think their control rate is substantially higher but I think their hypopituitarism rate is something on the order of three times what you presented. I suspect that if you tried to improve the remission rate you would have with it an increased associated hypopituitary rate.

Dr. Levin.   I think in continuity with Glenn's remarks, our center has a different approach than the other centers in that we are involved for at least the first 3 years in the patient's endocrine care and in the patient's primary care. For those 2 or 3 years we usually handle all their endocrine problems and some of their actual general medical problems, and we get to see them and care for some of their symptoms which are referable occasionally to pituitary insufficiency. I believe to make the diagnosis of absence or presence of pituitary insufficiency an insulin hypoglycemia test should be done. Dr. Kjellberg, do you do these on your patients?

Dr. Kjellberg.   This is done when the patient is in our endocrine unit. Many of our patients are followed from the source of referral.

Dr. Levin.   I think if these are done on patients you will reveal the fact that there are a percentage of patients who are totally asymptomatic and who have normal baseline values but have no evidence of reserve. Therefore these reserve tests as they are done will bring out more of the insufficiency of the ability to secrete ACTH. The other question I had and which I will direct to Dr. Sheline and Dr. Kramer is in reference to cysts. I am quite interested in these cysts. Are they cysts in the general pathologic definition of it, are they lined with epithelium, or are they lined with fibrous tissue? The epithelium would imply to me that there is some sort of congenital problem whereas a fibrous tissue lining really is not strictly a cyst and this would mean that the tumor had somehow grown and had a small infarction at one time. Do you have any information regarding this, that is, the histology of such cysts and what their etiology is? Are there any patients with pituitary tumors who should not have a pneumoencephalogram, and who should not even have any therapy? This includes the old and debilitated. Is it now accepted that all patients who are not extremely debilitated and who have a pituitary tumor or an enlarged sella should have a pneumoencephalogram and some form of therapy?

Dr. Seydel.   Before having answers to these questions, I would like to ask our neurosurgeon on the afternoon speaker list, Dr. Kjellberg, to give his explanation.

Dr. Kjellberg.   When we began trying to record our data, we found in many instances that to make suitable comparisons with other data was difficult. And I think that one of the things that we have come to have is a definite feeling that not only the record of the growth hormone is important, but you have to be more specific about the relationship of the clinical response, both in terms of the quality of the response and the duration. And I would favor what has been suggested earlier that we have something that is more uniform in reporting because I suspect the data exists, but from the reports of Dr. Kramer and Dr. Sheline I can't tell enough about the quality of the clinical response. I have found enough instances of reports of an occasional growth hormone level to be misleading but I would be grateful for an amplification of the clinical data in some quantitative way on the radiation-treated cases. I think also the interval of response is important as was emphasized by Dr. Levin. These patients should not continue to be very active acromegalics while they evolve the secondary features of the disease. The enlargement of the hands and the facial features is really not very important. Most of these people are not as bothered by it as by the evolution of cardiomyopathy, diabetes, and so forth. This is what makes these people sick and that's what puts them in the grave. And they should not wait around for years for that to happen. A relatively early prompt reduction of growth hormone associated with a very clear-cut clinical and endocrinological change is an imperative feature for the assessment of the response of any kind of therapy, and this should not be left as an open or unclear issue in the evaluation.

And it has been our view that perhaps if what I reported was my own personal experience. In that sense I am not for or against one form of therapy or the other, but we have made the judgements on what forms of therapy are available in individual cases on our own specific experience. My view is that the principal object of any form of therapy is to avoid mortality and that is a primary consideration. The other object, of course, is to get the result you are going for because if it doesn't produce the result then you shouldn't have either wasted the patient's time or exposed them to the risk.

Dr. Kramer.   I think Dr. Kjellberg has discussed this once or twice before. I think what he says is absolutely true. If we could come up with some kind of standard evaluation of these patients it would make everybody's life a great deal easier. Until we do that I think there has to be some kind of a belief in what is being reported. I think if we report that we have 25 out of 29 acromegalics who have shown an excellent clinical response, it also means that these people have returned to a normal existence where they have been able to work and so on. As far as the growth hormone levels are concerned, I think almost everybody who follows these cases now does multiple determinations, as we follow the patients, and certainly I think that probably they are a little more valid if they are done in the same lab and by the same people than if they are done from a distance. So it seems to me that the fact that these patients have lost their acromegalic features, that have lost their orthopedic problems, the carpal tunnel syndromes, and so on is indicative of the fact that the disease indeed has been arrested.

As I had mentioned earlier where we have seen a failure of growth hormone reduction we have also had clinical evidence of recurrence. And I think those two go hand in hand. With regard to the cysts, as Dr. Levin probably knows, by the time this material reaches the pathological laboratory it's rather hard to reconstitute the shape of the tumor because you get the fluid and then you get a bit of cyst wall and I have no idea what constitutes the cyst wall in these patients. I have a very good idea in craniopharyngiomas but that's another subject. So I can't answer that and as regards the air studies in investigation of patients with chromophobe adenomas, it depends what you are going to do. I would imagine that nobody who is going to operate on these patients would want to do that without at least an arteriogram because I have known carotid artery aneurysms in the way and that is a very unhealthy situation. And if you are going to irradiate them, then I would want an air study because I think we have to know what we are dealing with, (a) that there is a tumor and (b) what the extent of the tumor is. Whether or not you should ever treat a chromophobe adenoma, I don't know, I personally don't believe that these patients ever become burnt out cases and I think Dr. Sheline has some evidence to show that these patients ultimately get into trouble.

Dr. Sheline.   My surgical colleagues frequently call me to surgery to show me down through a little hole and I see them removing bits and pieces, and most of it is in the jar underneath the operating table along with the rest of the blood.

The question of time, I really don't know the importance of this. I think in principle the sooner one controls any disease probably the better. However, many of these patients if not most of them have histories that extend from 5 to 10 or 15 or 30 years, and whether a year or two longer makes any appreciable difference I think would be impossible to show because I think the only way to show this is in mortality and followup and I don't think we have that data.

In reviewing our case material a few years ago, I ran into a number of cases in which the presumptive diagnosis of a chromophobe adenoma had been made. There was no evidence of endocrinologic disturbance excepting I think that some of them may have had some mild hypopituitarism, but basically this was a group of patients in which a skull x-ray for some reason or another had shown an enlarged and eroded sella, and also again for some reason or another the patient had never been treated. Now you will see there are some 16 patients here; they had never been seen after the initial visit and this is simply a record of what happened to them in the subsequent years. Of the 16, you will note that for one reason or another 14 were ultimately treated. Larger sellas were noted on follow-up skull films up to periods extending up to 15 years. A group of 8 initially had field defects. Two increased their field defects, and 3 enlarged their sellae. In the group of 8 that initially had no field defects from periods of 6 months to 8 years, 5 had a field defect later. The end result was that 14 of the 16 ended up in surgery, and 7 of the 14 ended up with either increased field defects over their initial time of observation or field defects which were not there initially. So I, as Dr. Kramer eluded to, would take a sort of a dim view of following these patients without doing something.

Dr. Kjellberg. Many pituitary lesions are cystic, but adenomatous cysts normally have scraps of solid tumor on the wall. In many instances, I believe you cannot make the diagnosis preoperatively of the nature of a cyst. We operated on a cyst about 1 year ago and it was an arachnoidal cyst. I think it is true that if they are cystic their responsiveness to radiation is rather less satisfactory, but if the presenting symptom is a field defect this is one of the reasons we favor getting at it with a transnasal operation. A transnasal operation is extremely benign in a cyst. Frontal craniotomy, under any circumstances, is several times more hazardous and more productive of morbidity and possibly mortality than a transnasal operation. A great deal of effort is worth making to avoid a transfrontal operation whenever possible.

Dr. Chang.   May I comment about cysts in pituitary adenomas. About 5 years ago I reviewed a series of 303 cases of chromophobe adenoma in our material and I found 18% contained cysts, the list varied from microscopic cysts to a large cyst up to 33 cc in volume. Most of this material identified by the pathologist contained an epithelial cell lining. So I think these are true cysts. At that time we reported a series and we make speculation that if a tumor contained cyst, probably it was going to be radioresistant and we did make a recommendation if the cystic type of a tumor probably should have surgery.

The Treatment of Metastatic Disease of the Nervous System by Radiation Therapy

Luther W. Brady, M.D.,

Professor and Chairman,
Department of Therapeutic
Radiology and Nuclear Medicine,
Hahnemann Medical College
and Hospital, Philadelphia,
Pennsylvania

John Antoniades, M.D.,

Associate Professor,
Department of Radiation Therapy
and Nuclear Medicine,
Hahnemann Medical College,
Philadelphia, Pennsylvania

S. Prasasvinichai, M.D.,

Assistant Professor,
Department of Radiation Therapy
and Nuclear Medicine,
Hahnemann Medical College,
Philadelphia, Pennsylvania

Richard J. Torpie, M.D.,

Assistant Professor,
Department of Radiation Therapy
and Nuclear Medicine,
Hahnemann Medical College,
Philadelphia, Pennsylvania

Sucha O. Asbell, M.D.,

Assistant Professor,
Department of Radiation Therapy
and Nuclear Medicine,
Hahnemann Medical College,
Philadelphia, Pennsylvania

John R. Glassburn, M.D.,

Assistant Professor,
Department of Radiation Therapy
and Nuclear Medicine,
Hahnemann Medical College,
Philadelphia, Pennsylvania

David Schatanoff, M.D.,

Assistant Professor,
Department of Radiation Therapy
and Nuclear Medicine,
Hahnemann Medical College,
Philadelphia, Pennsylvania

Elliott L. Mancall, M.D.,

Professor of Medicine,
Director, Division of Neurology,
Hahnemann Medical College,
Philadelphia, Pennsylvania

The incidence of metastatic disease of the central nervous system represents 1–5% of all cases of cancer.[13] The incidence of metastatic intracranial disease is increasing steadily although it remains a rarity in children. The primary sites of malignancies metastasizing to the central nervous system vary from time to time and from one part of the world to another. In the United States, about 11,000 patients are said to be affected by this disease annually, although the number may be much higher.[3, 8, 14, 27] The common and primary sites are: bronchus (31–34%), breast (13–39%), gastrointestinal tract (16%), kidney (8%), skin (7%), and thyroid (4%). Metastatic disease to the central nervous system accounts for 4.1–26.3% of all central nervous system tumors. Metastases to the central nervous system are multiple in 70% of patients afflicted and are likely to coexist with metastases to other sites.

Metastases occur in a course of malignancy and may be of three essential types: (1) metachronous metastases where the primary lesion has been successfully controlled and months to years later, a focus is found at a distant site (7–14% of all brain metastases); (2) precocious metastases where the metastatic lesion is the first sign of cancer with no detectable evidence of a primary source (5–10% of all brain metastases); and (3) synchronous metastases where a solitary metastatic lesion and a defined primary cancer are presented simultaneously (80–85% of all brain metastases).[33]

The frequency of solitary metastases to the brain and central nervous system varies considerably. They are a function of the type of experience being analyzed whether surgical or necropsy. Metastases to the central nervous system are multiple in the majority of cases, but do occur as a solitary focus in 30–36% of cases. Only 7–14% are without associated extracranial metastatic disease.

Metastatic malignant tumors involving the spinal cord are generally extradural in character. They are generally similar in type to those occurring within the brain, but differ in incidence, a reflection of the differences in the quantity of medullary tissue in cord coverings.

The purpose of this presentation is to discuss the treatment programs to be employed in intracranial metastatic neoplasia and in metastatic spinal cord tumors.

INTRACRANIAL METASTATIC NEOPLASMS

Treatment of this relatively common neurological disorder is unfortunately all too often marked by frustration and resignation on the part of all concerned. Surgical management of cerebral metastases is for the most part, disappointing, but some modification on the outlook based on therapy with radiation techniques is appropriate. Radiation therapy alone is preferable to surgery in the management of metastatic disease to the brain when the primary neoplasm is not under control, when there are widespread metastases elsewhere in the body, or where multiple intracranial lesions are manifest, particularly if the tumor has been demonstrated to be radiosensitive. It is insufficiently appreciated that radiation therapy, in fact, may be associated with significant and, at times, remarkable relief of signs and symptoms in many cases[8, 10, 13-15, 23, 27, 28, 30, 31, 39, 41.] Support of this contention emerges from an in-depth study of the ma-

This study was supported by Public Health Services Research Grants No. 1 R10 CA12252 and No. 1 R10 CA12478 from the National Cancer Institute, by Public Health Services Training Grant No. T01 CA05185 from the National Cancer Institute, by the Friends of the Radiation Therapy Center, and by the Alperin Foundation.

terial seen at the Hahnemann Medical College and Hospital representing the experience of a clinical team dealing with problems of metastatic intracranial malignancy. The widespread persistence of a nihilistic attitude toward the treatment of cerebral metastasis by radiation technique is inappropriate.

In the review of 229 consecutive patients with intracranial metastatic disease seen from 1961 to 1972, patients ranged from 2 to 80 years of age, with a median of 55 years. There were 163 males and 66 females, with 195 of the patients being white and 34 black. The most common primary site was the lung, representing 147 patients (64.2%). About 14% of the patients had primary site from the breast. The gastrointestinal and genitourinary tract accounted for many of the remainder, with 7.4% having lymphomatous disease or multiple myeloma (Table 1).

The most commonly encountered presenting symptoms were those of hemiparesis or hemiplegia, with headache, dizziness, and seizures being common (Table 2). The symptoms in general reflected the location of the tumor. The relative incidence of metastasis varied from 78% in the cerebrum to 5% in the cerebellum and 17% in the multiple sites. Kindt[20] and Allen[2] have pointed out a definite predilection for metastases to lodge along the posterior aspect of the Rolandic fissure in the region of the junction of the temporal, parietal, and occipital lobes. In large measure, the tumors were located within the distribution of the middle cerebral artery with the possible explanation that the location was related to the principals of blood flow in the arteries. In general, there was no preponderance of lesions either to the right or the left side.

TABLE 1.   INTRACRANIAL METASTATIC MALIGNANCY: SITE OF THE PRIMARY LESION (1961–1972)

	No. Patients	Percent
Lung (squamous cell or undifferentiated carcinoma)	147	64.2
Breast (adenocarcinoma)	33	14.4
Leukemia	10	4.4
Multiple myeloma	2	0.9
Giant follicular lymphoma	1	0.4
Hodgkin's disease	3	1.3
Reticulum cell sarcoma	1	0.4
Retromolar (squamous cell carcinoma)	1	0.4
Nasopharynx (squamous cell carcinoma)	4	1.9
Larynx (squamous cell carcinoma)	1	0.4
Gastrointestinal (esophagus, 1 squamous cell carcinoma; stomach, 2; colon, 4; rectum, 2 adenocarcinoma)	10	4.4
Kidney (adenocarcinoma)	4	1.8
Prostate (adenocarcinoma)	3	1.3
Mesothelioma	1	0.4
Melanoma	2	0.9
Unknown	6	2.6
Total	229	100.0

TABLE 2. INTRACRANIAL METASTATIC MALIGNANCY:
PRESENTING SYMPTOMS AND SIGNS IN
229 PATIENTS (1961–1972)

	No. Patients	Percent
Hemiparesis and hemiplegia	92	40
Headache	73	32
Dizziness and vertigo	27	12
Convulsions	32	14
Memory loss	39	17
Visual disturbance	25	11

The diagnosis was established on the basis of a careful history and neurological examination, with diagnostic studies being carried out including roentgenograms of the skull in all cases (these being positive in terms of displacement of the pineal gland or indirect evidence of increased intracranial pressure in only 33 patients), brain scans being performed in 208 patients with 181 demonstrating positive results, and arteriograms or ventriculograms being performed in 61 patients with 49 being interpreted as positive (Table 3).

A relatively small proportion of patients demonstrated multiple lesions and this may simply reflect the fact that the data are based on observations *intra vitam*. One would expect a much higher incidence of multiple lesions if the brains themselves were to be examined pathologically, since all lesions which do not manifest clinically or radiographically are frequently evident at necropsy.

TABLE 3. INTRACRANIAL
METASTATIC
MALIGNANCY: LOCATION
OF DOMINANT
METASTASIS AS
DETERMINED BY BRAIN
SCAN TECHNIQUES
(1961–1972)

	No. Patients	Percent
Parietal	61	31
Frontal	41	21
Frontoparietal	22	11
Temporal	14	7
Cerebellum	10	5
Parieto-occipital	8	4
Parietotemporal	8	4
Multiple	33	17
Total	197	100

The treatment program is carried out on all patients with external radiation therapy with the intent to irradiate the entire brain through two parallel opposed fields. This approach was adopted in view of the hematogenous dissemination of the disease and the anticipated multiplicity of the intracerebral lesions. The calculated tumor dose was estimated at the midplane of the brain and was 4000 rads in a median elapsed time of 28 days. Supervoltage radiation therapy techniques were utilized in the majority of patients and 185 patients received high-dose steroid therapy during the course of radiation therapy. No patient required interruption of treatment due to "radiation edema" and all exhibited epilation at the completion of treatment, but the hair regrew in the survivors in 6 months.

Thirteen patients required a second course of radiation therapy because of recurrence of symptoms, the dose level being a median calculated tumor dose of 2500 rads in a median elapsed time of 3 weeks.

Craniotomy was carried out in 21 patients prior to the institution of radiation therapy, but in no instance was tumor removal judged to be complete.

The median survival of the 198 patients who completed the projected course of radiation therapy for intracranial metastatic disease was 4.5 months from the day of completion of their radiation therapy. Twenty-seven patients died during radiation therapy, but in no instance could death be attributed directly to the radiation therapy. An excellent response to treatment, defined as complete disappearance of symptoms with the patient being capable both intellectually and physically of resuming his former occupation was achieved by 66 patients with a median survival in this group of 7 months (Table 4). A good response was defined as a good return of function but with some limitations in activity and minimal neurological deficit. In this category, 63 patients were identified and had a median survival of 6 months. A fair response to treatment was characterized by persistent, debilitating symptoms albeit with some return of function. Thirty-seven patients exhibited in this degree of response with a median survival of 2.0 months. A persistent and incapacitating deficit but with minimal improvement characterized a poor response to treatment. Sixteen patients had such a poor response, and their median survival was 2 months. Sixteen patients failed to improve in any recognizable respect. The best median survivals were those obtained in

TABLE 4. INTRACRANIAL METASTATIC
MALIGNANCY: MEDIAN
SURVIVAL AFTER COMPLETION
OF TREATMENT ACCORDING TO
RESPONSE (1961–1972)

	No. Patients	Median survival (months)
Excellent	66	7.0 (1–38)
Good	63	6.0 (2–24)
Fair	37	2.0 (1–21)
Poor	16	2.0 (1–8)
None	16	1.0
Total	198	4.5

carcinoma of the breast and carcinoma of the rectum (Table 5). Of the 185 patients who were given high-dose steroid therapy, the median survival was 6 months compared with the overall median survival of the entire group of 4.5 months.[21]

The radiation therapist encounters a high proportion of patients who develop metastatic deposits in the central nervous system for whom treatment is deemed appropriate. The symptoms caused by the cerebral metastases themselves, the general condition of the patient, the number and size of other metastases, the site and histological nature of the primary lesion, and previous treatment are all relevant factors in considering the most advisable form of treatment.

Our present experience would suggest that although in an unselected series of cases, radiation therapy cannot result in cure, good or excellent palliative results may be obtained in a remarkably high proportion of cases. The ultimate effect with regard to prolongation of life may be negligible, since the average duration of life in untreated cases approximates 3 months versus 4.5 months in the treated group. Unfortunately, neither the degree nor the duration of relief of symptoms is predictable in an individual patient, and even in some apparently hopeless cases, unexpectedly good to excellent results have been obtained, in some instances lasting as long as 38 months. In 176 patients there was no clinical evidence of regrowth of the tumor involving the brain. These data would thus favor the utilization of radiation therapy in patients with metastatic intracranial deposits, particularly those considered not suitable for definitive neurosurgical intervention, but whose death from generalized disease is not imminent.

The Radiation Therapy Oncology Group has undertaken the evaluation of the most appropriate treatment program from a radiation therapy point of view in the management of intracranial metastatic disease. The data accumulated thus far indicate that there is no significant difference in survival among the fractionation–protraction techniques being employed, namely, 3000 rads to the midplane of the brain in 15 elapsed days, 4000 rads to the midplane of the brain in 15 elapsed days, or 4000 rads to the midplane of the brain in 20 elapsed days using parallel opposed fields and supervoltage techniques. The addition of steroids to the treatment program did seem to effect a prompt improvement (Table 6).[22]

From the data in this study, a new protocol for the treatment of brain metastasis was initiated on November 1, 1973 to evaluate 2000 rads to the midplane of the brain in 5 elapsed days, 3000 rads to the midplane of the brain in 10 elapsed days, and 4000 rads to the midplane of the brain in 15 elapsed days. If the treatment programs in a shorter

TABLE 5.   INTRACRANIAL METASTATIC
           MALIGNANCY: MEDIAN SURVIVAL
           AFTER COMPLETION OF TREATMENT
           ACCORDING TO PRIMARY SITE
           (1961–1972)

Primary Site	Median survival (months)
Lung	4.2
Breast	8.0
Other	5

TABLE 6.   INTRACRANIAL   METASTATIC   MALIGNANCY   RTOG   STUDY
(SEPT. 1973) 804 PATIENTS

Tumor Dose (rads)	Elapsed Days	NSD (rets)	Median Survival (weeks)
3000	10	1300	15.4
3000	15	1130	14.8
4000	15	1500	13.2
4000	20	1360	12.9

period of time prove to be as effective as the higher dosages in a longer period of time, the saving in time and effort will be considerable.

On the basis of these data, palliative radiation therapy for intracranial metastases appears justified. The relief of symptoms and the lessening of disability afford major benefit in the terminal care of such patients.

METASTATIC SPINAL CORD TUMORS

In reviewing the literature, the value of radiation therapy for management of metastatic spinal cord tumors is difficult to assess.[1, 4-8, 11, 12, 16-19, 24-26, 29, 34-38, 40] Intramedullary metastasis to the spinal cord from distant malignant tumors is rare, with only 3 cases reported in the literature.[8, 11] Extramedullary metastatic lesions to the spinal cord are not uncommon. The spinal cord may be damaged by such metastatic lesions by direct infiltration, by pressure secondary to vertebral collapse, or by pressure secondary to vascular occlusion produced by the metastatic lesion.[6] The diagnosis is established by a careful history and neurological examination, roentgenograms of the spine (about 50% of patients will demonstrate bone involvement), and myelography.[7, 12, 25] There is a paucity of information in the literature regarding the correlation of prognosis to treatment in cases treated by surgery alone or a combination of surgery and radiation therapy.

The experience of the Hahnemann Medical College and Hospital relates to 133 patients with the diagnosis of metastatic spinal cord tumor seen from 1958 through 1972. Many different histological cell types were represented in the series, but the most common ones encountered were metastatic lesions from the lung, breast, and lymphomas and myelomas (Table 7). The incidence was about 0.2–4% of the total number of cases seen with each tumor type.

The signs and symptoms of neurological involvement fell into three groups: sensory, motor, and sphincter involvement. Sensory symptoms consisted of numbness and radicular pain. Motor symptoms were those of muscular weakness or paralysis of the extremities. The sphincteric symptoms were urinary hesitancy or frequency progressing to complete retention, or bowel involvement in the form of constipation progressing to obstipation. In careful review of the patient's history, the most common complaint leading to medical care was weakness of the lower extremities, although 90% of the patients studied revealed sensory involvement as their first neurologic deficit. About 5% of the patients showed involvement of the motor system as their first sign and only 1 patient had sphincteric involvement as the only sign of spinal cord involvement. The

TABLE 7. PRIMARY LESIONS IN METASTATIC SPINAL CORD TUMORS

	No. Cases (Percent of Cases in Each Disease Category)	Total No. New Cases Seen with Each Diagnosis 1958–1972
Lung	39 (3.6)	1090
Breast	37 (3.4)	1103
Lymphoma and myeloma	25 (3.8)	650
Gastrointestinal (colon and stomach)	6 (0.9)	689
Urinary Tract	6 (1.8)	340
Reproductive (uterus, ovary, and cervix)	5 (0.2)	1960
Miscellaneous (parotid, thyroid, etc.)	5	—
Unknown	10	—
Total	133	

average duration of sensory symptoms was 42 days, motor signs 17 days, and sphincteric findings 3 days (Table 8). The level of metastatic involvement was most commonly encountered in the cauda equina, being represented by 38.4% of the cases. The level was from T-5 to L-1 in 22.5% of the patients and from T-1 to T-4 in 29.3% of the patients, and cervical involvement was demonstrated in 9.8% (Table 9). The tumor level was established by a careful history, a careful neurological examination, and roentgenograms of the spine, with confirmation being established by myelography.

In the experience being recorded, surgery was the primary means of therapy in the early years. It was not until 1960 that a well-defined approach to the problem of metastatic carcinoma involving the spinal cord was initiated. At that point, it was decided that when pressure symptoms developed and the position of the defect could be established, immediate laminectomy was to be performed to relieve pressure and lessen the chances of permanent cord damage. In all instances, radiation therapy was to follow. The majority of the patients have been treated by such an approach to the problem. It was also felt that immediate decompression was imperative when extradural pressure on the cord was due to collapse of a vertebral body that contained

TABLE 8. METASTATIC SPINAL CORD TUMORS: DURATION OF SYMPTOMS PRIOR TO TREATMENT

Symptoms	Extremes	Average (days)
Sensory	1 day to 1 year	42
Motor	1 day to 6 months	17
Sphincter	1 hour to 1 month	3

TABLE 9. METASTATIC SPINAL CORD
TUMORS: DISTRIBUTION OF THE
LEVEL OF INVOLVEMENT

Level	No. Patients	Percent
C-1 to C-7	13	9.8
T-1 to T-4	39	29.3
T-5 to L-1	30	22.5
Cauda equina	51	38.4
Total	133	100.0

metastases, and in such instances radiation therapy was to follow. In the early years, patients were occasionally treated with minimal symptoms by either surgery or radiation therapy.

Postoperatively the area of involvement was irradiated using radiation therapy techniques with a median dosage of 3500–4000 rads delivered at depth in a median time of 25–30 elapsed days. Radiation therapy was begun within the first 2–3 days following decompression in those patients operated or immediately in those who were treated exclusively by radiation techniques. The fields chosen were wide enough to encompass the cord with a wide margin above and below the demonstrated defect. No areas of involvement required retreatment. Supplementary data accumulated as a consequence of the procedure represented exploration above and below the point of block in order to determine the presence of single or multiple lesions involving the cord. When lesions could be demonstrated in multiple sites, adequate fields needed to be chosen in order to encompass those areas.

The return of motor function as related to the level of cord involvement was analyzed in detail (Table 10). The best results were obtained in those patients when both surgery and radiation therapy were employed as the technique for the management of the problem.

TABLE 10. METASTATIC SPINAL CORD TUMORS:
RETURN OF MOTOR FUNCTION
RELATED TO THE CORD LEVEL
OF METASTASIS

	Number of Treated Patients Responding		
Level	Surgery	Surgery and Radiation	Radiation
C-1 to C-7	0 of 3	6 of 8	1 of 2
T-1 to T-4	0 of 4	20 of 33	1 of 2
T-5 to L-1	3 of 8	9 of 15	5 of 7
Cauda equina	4 of 9	20 of 34	2 of 8

TABLE 11. METASTATIC SPINAL CORD TUMORS: RETURN OF MOTOR FUNCTION RELATED TO THE DEGREE OF PARESIS

Degree of Paresis	Number of Treated Patients Responding		
	Surgery	Surgery and Radiation	Radiation
Marked	1 of 14	14 of 38	3 of 10
Moderate	4 of 8	31 of 42	2 of 4
Mild	2 of 2	10 of 10	4 of 5

Muscle weakness in the lower extremities was classified as mild, moderate, or marked. Mild paresis occurred in those patients who had clinically demonstrable weakness but were still able to ambulate unassisted. Moderate paresis indicated that the patients required assistance to ambulate. Marked paresis referred to complete paralysis or paresis to such a degree that the patients were unable to support their body weight. Return of motor function was studied in relation to the degree of paresis and it was found that the prognosis corresponded directly to the degree of paresis (Table 11). Of those patients with moderate paresis, 74% showed recovery as compared with only 37% of the cases with marked paresis when treated by combination of surgery and radiation therapy. The poorest response was seen in those patients treated by surgery alone or by radiation therapy alone. The longer the duration of involvement, the less favorable the prognosis. It is also evident that the shorter the interval between the onset of symptoms and the institution of therapy, the more likely that function will return.

The median survival in the patients with metastatic carcinoma of the lung was 87 days, whereas for those with metastatic carcinoma of the breast, the median survival was 7 months and in those with lymphoma or myeloma, 12 months (Table 12).

The present experience confirms the fact, as demonstrated by others,[4, 5, 38] that primary carcinoma of the lung has a high potential for metastasizing to the epidural space of the spinal cord. Carcinoma of the breast has also been reported to be a common primary lesion for epidural metastases and Hodgkin's disease produces compression of the spinal cord in about 4% of patients.[16, 18, 34] The rate of progression of neurological deficit and its duration are related to the return of motor function

TABLE 12. METASTATIC SPINAL CORD TUMORS: SURVIVAL IN EACH TUMOR TYPE FOLLOWING TREATMENT

Tumor Type	No. Patients	Median Survival (Range)
Lung	39	87 days (9-167 days)
Breast	37	7 months (10 days to 6 years)
Lymphoma and myeloma	25	12 months (2 months to 5 years)

TABLE 13. METASTATIC SPINAL CORD TUMORS:
DURATION OF SYMPTOMS RELATED TO
RETURN OF FUNCTION FOLLOWING
TREATMENT

Return of Function	Average Duration of Symptoms (days)		
	Sensory	Motor	Sphincter
Good	29	16	1
None	42	22	4

following treatment (Table 13). The more rapid the progression and the longer the deficit remains untreated, the less favorable is the prognosis. These findings are in agreement with those of Tarlov.[36] Improvement in sensory deficit was noted in all patients regardless of treatment. The degree of paresis prior to surgery or radiation therapy or both is closely related to the return of motor function. Similar results have been reported by Mullan and Evans.[26] The importance of early diagnosis and treatment in cases of metastatic extramedullary spinal cord tumors has been stressed by other authors[5, 7, 26, 29, 36, 37] and is supported by our findings. The presence of sphincteric involvement was a less favorable prognostic sign. In the present series, patients with sphincteric involvement for more than 1 day showed no recovery regardless of the mode of treatment. The three groups of symptoms may serve as an index to the rapidity of progression of neurological deficit. The interval between motor and sphincteric involvement is much shorter in patients showing no recovery as compared with patients who have good motor return.

Tarlov[37] and Torma[38] demonstrated that interference with vascular supply is of more significance in causing neurologic deficit than direct pressure alone. The thoracic cord segment between T-1 and T-4, ventrally and dorsally, is considered to be the most susceptible to vascular insult by virtue of the anatomical arrangement of the vascular supply in this area of the spinal cord.[25] Less favorable results in cases with involvement at this level were noted when compared with cases involving the other segments of the spinal cord regardless of the tumor type or the mode of therapy.

From careful evaluation of the present series, the role of radiation therapy in conjunction with surgery is supported by the evidence of the results obtained.

SUMMARY

Metastases to the brain are usually multiple, and treatment, if indicated, should include the entire brain. Significant improvement in an incapacitating disability can be achieved by prompt and effectively managed radiation therapy.

In the management of metastatic disease to the central nervous system, survival figures are not especially meaningful. These patients should be treated aggressively for relief of distressing symptoms and not for cure or increased longevity.

In the management of epidural spinal cord metastases, prompt diagnosis is mandatory, and definitive, although palliative, treatment should be promptly instituted. If at the time of diagnosis, there is progressive or even unmeasured neurological deficit, surgical decompression should precede the irradiation to avoid cord damage from pressure of vascular insufficiency.

Aggressive radiation therapy is justified and the relief of symptoms and lessening of disability do afford major benefit in the terminal care of such patients.

REFERENCES

1. Alexander, E., Jr., Davis, C. H., Jr., and Fields, C. H., Jr.: Metastatic Lesions of Vertebra Column Causing Cord Compression. *Neurology* **6**:103–109 (January) (1956).

2. Allen, M. B., Jr., Dick, D. A., and Hightower, S. S.: The Value and Limitations of Brain Scanning, A Review of 401 Consecutive Cases. *Clin. Radiol.* **18**:19–27 (1967).

3. Aronson, S. M., Garcia, J. H., and Aronson, B. E.: Metastatic Neoplasms of the Brain: Their Frequency in Relation to Age. *Cancer* **17**:558–563 (1964).

4. Arseni, C. N., Simionescu, M. D., and Horwath, L.: Tumors of the Spine. *Acta Psychiat. Scand.* **34**:398–410 (1959).

5. Barron, K. D., Hirano, A., Araki, S., and Terry, R. D.: Experience with Metastatic Neoplasms Involving the Spinal Cord. *Neurology* **9**:91–106 (January 1959).

6. Batson, O. V.: Role of Vertebral Veins in Metastatic Processes. *Ann. Internal Med.* **16**:38–45 (January 1942).

7. Botterell, E. H., and Fitzgerald, G. W.: Spinal Cord Compression Produced by Extradural Malignant Tumors: Early Recognition, Treatment and Results. *Can. Med. Assoc. J.* **80**:791–795 (May 15, 1959).

8. Bouchard, J.: Central Nervous System. In Fletcher, G. H., Ed., *Textbook of Radiotherapy*, Lea & Febiger, Philadelphia, 1966, pp. 247–300.

9. Bouchard, J.: Radiation Therapy of Metastatic Intracranial Tumors. In Gletcher, G. H., Ed., *Radiation Therapy of Tumors and Diseases of the Nervous System*, Lea & Febiger, Philadelphia, 1966, pp. 167–180.

10. Bowen, R., Jr., Knapp, J. R., and Collins, V. P.: Radiotherapy of Cerebral Metastases. *Texas State J. Med.* **61**:894–898 (1965).

11. Cantor, M. B., and Stein, J. M.: Intramedullary Spinal Cord Metastasis. *J. Nervous Mental Disease* **115**:351–355 (April) (1952).

12. Chambers, W. R.: Intraspinal Tumors: A Difficult Diagnosis. *Amer. J. Surg.* **87**:824–829 (June) (1954).

13. Chao, J., Phillips, R., and Nickson, J. J.: Roentgen-Ray Therapy of Cerebral Metastases. *Cancer* **7**:682–689 (1954).

14. Chason, J. L., Walker, F. B., and Landers, J. W.: Metastatic Carcinoma in the Central Nervous System and Dorsal Root Ganglia. *Cancer* **16**:781–787 (1963).

15. Chu, F. C., and Hilaris, B. B.: Value of Radiation Therapy in the Management of Intracranial Metastases. *Cancer* **14**:577–581 (1961).

16. Diamond, H. D.: Hodgkin's Disease: Neurologic Sequelae. *Missouri Med.* **54**:945–955 (October 1957).

17. Elsberg, C. A.: *Surgical Diseases of the Spinal Cord, Membranes and Nerve Roots*, Paul B. Hoeber, Medical Book Dept., Harper and Row, New York, 1941, p. 501.

18. Jelliffe, A. M., and Thomson, A. D.: The Prognosis in Hodgkin's Disease. *Brit. J. Cancer* **9**:21–36 (March 1955).

19. Kennedy, J. C. and Stern, W. E.: Metastatic Compression of the Spinal Cord. *Amer. J. Surg.* **104**:155–168 (August 1962).

20. Kindt, G. W.: The Pattern of Location of Cerebral Metastatic Tumors. *J. Neurosurg.* **21**:54–57 (1964).

21. King, D. F., Moon, W. J., and Brown, N.: Corticosteroid Drugs in the Management of Primary and Secondary Malignant Cerebral Tumors. *Med. J. Australia* **2**:878–881 (1965).

22. Kramer, S.: Personal communication, 1973.

23. Lang, E. F., and Slater, J.: Metastatic Brain Tumors—Results of Surgical and Nonsurgical Treatment. *Surg. Clin. North Amer.* **44**:865–872 (1964).

24. Love, J. G., Miller, R. H., and Keenohan, J. W.: Lymphomas of the Spinal Cord Epidural Space. *Arch. Surg.* **69**:66–76 (July 1954).

25. McAlhany, H. J. and Netsky, M. G.: Compression of the Spinal Cord by Extramedullary Neoplasms: A Clinical and Pathological Study. *J. Neuropath. Exptl. Neurol.* **14**:276–287 (July 1955).

26. Mullan, J. and Evans, J. P.: Neoplastic Diseases of the Spinal Extradural Space: A Review of 50 Cases. *Arch. Surg.* **74**:900–999 (June 1957).

27. Murphy, W.: *Radiation Therapy,* W. Saunders, Philadelphia, 1967, pp. 399–400.

28. O'Connell, J. E.: The Place of Surgery in Intracranial Metastatic Malignant Disease. *Proc. Royal Soc. Med.* **57**:1159–1164 (1964).

29. Perse, D. M.: Treatment of Metastatic Extradural Spinal Cord Tumors. *Cancer* **11**:214–231 (1958).

30. Pool, J. L., Ransohoff, J., and Cornell, J. W.: The Treatment of Malignant Brain Tumors, Primary and Metastatic. *N.Y. J. Med.* **57**:3983–3988 (1957).

31. Richards, P., and McKissock, W.: Intracranial Metastases. *Brit. Med. J.* **1**:15–18 (1963).

32. Rogers, L.: Malignant Spinal Cord Tumors and Epidural Space. *Brit. J. Surg.* **45**:416–422 (April 1958).

33. Rubin, P., and Green, J.: *Solitary Metastases,* Charles C. Thomas, Springfield, Illinois, pp. 82–105.

34. Smith, M. J., and Stenstrom, K. W.: Compression of the Spinal Cord Caused by Hodgkin's Disease. *Radiology* **51**:77–84 (July 1958).

35. Spurling, R. G.: *Lesions of the Cervical Intervertebral Disc,* Charles C. Thomas, Springfield, Illinois, 1958.

36. Tarlov, I. M.: Spinal Cord Compression Studies: III. Time Limits for Recovery After Gradual Compression in Dogs. *Arch. Neurol. Psychiat.* **71**:588–597 (May 1954).

37. Tarlov, I. M., and Herj, E.: Spinal Cord Compression Studies: IV, Outlook with Complete Paralysis in Man. *Arch. Neurol. Psychiat.* **72**:43–59 (July 1954).

38. Torma, T.: Malignant Tumors of the Spine and the Extradural Space. *Acta Chir. Scand, Suppl.* **225,** 1–176 (May 1957).

39. Vieth, R. G., and Odom, G. L.: Intracranial Metastases and Their Neurosurgical Treatment. *J. Neurosurg.* *323*:375–383, (1965).

40. Wild, W., and Porter, R.: Metastatic Epidural Tumors of the Spine. *Arch. Surg.* **87**:835–830 (Nov 1963).

41. Windeyer, B.: Metastases in the Central Nervous System: Treatment by Radiotherapy and Chemotherapy. *Proc. Royal Soc. Med.* **57**:1153–1159, (1964).

Discussion

Dr. Kjellberg.   Have you considered chemotherapy in these patients?

Dr. Brady.   The problem with the utilization of chemotherapy in the management of brain metastasis I think is really illustrated by the fact that the results of treatment are not anywhere near the results that you can get from radiation therapy. One does not achieve the concentration of drug in order to effect prompt specific relief that you can get from radiation techniques. I think the same probably applies to spinal cord and epidural disease, although we have patients in our experience who have been treated by chemotherapy alone and who have never been irradiated, primarily prostate lesions, and who have done very well for very long periods of time. So I think there are exceptions in the cord. I don't think there are exceptions in the brain.

Index